C000260569

The
Phantom
Museum

The Phantom Museum

*and Henry Wellcome's
Collection of Medical Curiosities*

by
Peter Blegvad
A. S. Byatt
Helen Cleary
Tobias Hill
Hari Kunzru
Gaby Wood

Edited and with an introduction by
Hildi Hawkins and Danielle Olsen

P

PROFILE BOOKS

First published in Great Britain in 2003 by
PROFILE BOOKS LTD
58a Hatton Garden
London EC1N 8LX
www.profilebooks.co.uk

in association with The Wellcome Trust

The Wellcome Trust is an independent research-funding charity, established under the will of Sir Henry Wellcome in 1936. Its mission is to foster and promote research with the aim of improving human and animal health. Its work covers four areas:

Knowledge – improving our understanding of human and animal biology in health and disease, and of the past and present role of medicine in society;
Resources – providing exceptional researchers with the infrastructure and career support they need to fulfil their potential;
Translation – ensuring maximum health benefits are gained from biomedical research;
Public engagement – raising awareness of the medical, ethical, social and cultural implications of biomedical science.

Introduction and this complete collection copyright © The Trustee of The Wellcome Trust, 2003

The individual essays or contributions in this collection are copyright of the author in each case, as listed below, and are published here for the first time.
'Milk' copyright © Peter Blegvad, 2003
'Body Art' copyright © A. S. Byatt, 2003
'The Venus Time of Year' copyright © Helen Cleary, 2003
'Impossible Things' copyright © Tobias Hill, 2003
'The Collected' copyright © Hari Kunzru, 2003
'Phantom Limbs' copyright © Gaby Wood, 2003

Copyright material from other sources is reproduced by permission and acknowledged on page 207.

Illustrations on pages 106, 109 (bottom), 110, 111, 113, 116, 117 (top and bottom), 123 (left), 130, 132, 134 (middle), 139 (bottom) copyright © Peter Blegvad, 2003. Photographs on pages 46, 48, 52–3, 58, 62, 66–7, 73 copyright © Hari Kunzru, 2003. All other illustrations copyright © The Wellcome Trust, 2003. All illustrations except those by Peter Blegvad listed above are reproduced by permission of The Wellcome Trust. Full details of Wellcome Trust images appear in 'Wellcome's Things' on page 193.

10 9 8 7 6 5 4 3 2 1

The moral right of the authors has been asserted.

All rights reserved. Without limiting the rights under copyright reserved above, no part of this publication may be reproduced, stored or introduced into a retrieval system, or transmitted, in any form or by any means (electronic, mechanical, photocopying, recording or otherwise), without the prior written permission of both the copyright owner and the publisher of this book.

A CIP catalogue record for this book is available from the British Library.

ISBN 1 86197 618 6

Editorial consultant: Paul Forty
Text and cover design: Rose Design
Printed and bound in Great Britain by St Edmundsbury Press, Bury St Edmunds

Contents

Introduction

My cane, my pocket change, this ring of keys,
the obedient lock, the belated notes,
the few days left to me will not find time
to read, the deck of cards, the table-top,
a book encrushed in its pages the withered
violet, monument to an afternoon
undoubtedly unforgettable, now forgotten,
the mirror in the west where a red sunrise
blazes its illusion. How many things,
files, doorsills, atlases, nails,
serve us like slaves who never say a word,
blind and so mysteriously reserved.
They will endure beyond our vanishing;
and they will never know that we have gone.

'Things' by Jorge Luis Borges

One of the most poignant aspects of the world of inanimate objects is their longevity. They endure, and we do not; they fail to recognise our passing – and, to make matters worse, they are unspeaking witnesses that can never tell us what they have seen, who made them and why, who used them and what for, and what they meant.

This book celebrates one of the twentieth century's least known but most mysterious of museum collections. Henry Solomon Wellcome (1853–1936), entrepreneur and businessman, co-founder of Burroughs Wellcome & Co., one of the first giant pharmaceutical companies, was also an archaeologist and philanthropist with an absorbing interest in what he called 'the great past'. His motive in building up one of the world's largest collections of objects – as a whole, it numbers more than one million separate items – was to demonstrate 'by means of objects... the actuality of every notable step in the evolution and progress from the first germ of life to the fully developed man of today'. His aim, in other words, was no less than to trace the history of the human body, in sickness and in health, throughout the whole broad sweep of history.

What were the things he used to illustrate the noble story he wished to tell? He and his agents scoured the whole of the British empire, then at its zenith, and beyond, for anything and everything that relates to the human body. The objects the collection contains range from the very old (Neolithic vessels and Graeco-Roman votive offerings) to the magical and religious (masks and amulets) and the scientific (surgical instruments and microscopes). Their number – thousands of spears, spectacles and pictures; hundreds of manuscripts, syringes and forceps; dozens upon dozens of snuffboxes, anatomical manikins and tattoos – testifies to the one-time ubiquity of what might otherwise be considered rare or arcane objects.

Now dispersed in collections throughout the world, from Australia to Zimbabwe, the Wellcome collection is a vast repository not only of objects, but of traces of physical sensations, ideas and emotions, a reliquary of thoughts and fragments of memory. The soft, fleeting and ungraspable stuff of life is conjured up by matter of an altogether different nature, now lying inert in anachronistic institutions and very slowly turning to dust. It is the residue of a noisy history whose hubbub – breathing, choking, coughing, sneezing, laughing, hiccuping, screaming – is at last stilled.

This book forms a companion volume to the catalogue of an exhibition on Henry Wellcome's collection held at the British Museum in the summer of 2003. The aim of the exhibition was to reunite a fraction of the collection back in one place. The exhibition catalogue endeavours to present the facts of the collection, exploring its objects through documents and physical evidence.[1] Here, in *The Phantom Museum*, the objects are investigated using a different method, that of the sympathetic imagination.

Although united by their place in Wellcome's collection, many of the objects he amassed are so mysterious as to be inscrutable. Their catalogue remains incomplete; but even the accretions of knowledge that accompany them sometimes awake suspicion. What should we make of the 'gall bladder, stuffed with rice' or the 'amulet for draining milk from cats'? Others are objects on the verge of annihilation: 'Human dust from vaults of St Martin in the Fields found by F. T. Buckland in 1859'. Some of the most mysterious objects now even lack the labels which might once have helped us to decipher them; their meanings have become impenetrable. All of these things have been witness to the lives of the people who have at some point lived alongside them, used them or had them used upon them. How, we wondered on embarking on this book, might we tap into this huge reservoir of lives, this susurrus of experiences, pick up on the faintest of echoes at the end of a long line of Chinese whispers?

Our method was simple. We invited our writers – selected because we felt their hearing might be relied upon to be exceptionally sharp; they would, we hoped, have a particular affinity both with this project and with the collection itself – to tour the biggest remaining group of Wellcome's things, which is housed in a storeroom in West London. We introduced them to the collection and suggested points of interest, but otherwise said as little as possible in order to allow the most direct contact with the objects themselves. And the rest – give or take some occasionally intense discussion – was up to them.

It is worth saying a word or two about the living conditions our objects currently find themselves in. Sequestered in the vaults of what was once the National Savings Bank, Blythe House in Hammersmith, they lie for

---

1 *Medicine Man: the Forgotten Museum of Henry Wellcome*, edited by Ken Arnold and Danielle Olsen, British Museum Press, 2003

the most part undisturbed and, as far as we know, mute, guarding their secrets. Dark, cool rooms line the long basement corridors, each crammed with objects and each with a different character. Objects are classified by room – Glassware, Oriental, Surgery – giving rise to a higgledy-piggledy arrangement in which snuffboxes rub shoulders with mourning jewellery, ear trumpets with dentist's chairs and anatomical models with human bones. This sense of disorientation, as well as the sheer iteration which was part of Wellcome's method for imposing order on his objects, has made its way into A. S. Byatt's description of the fictional Eli Pettifer collection in the first story of the book, 'Body Art':

> There were bottles – ancient tear-bottles, ornate pharmacy bottles in pale rose with gilded letters, preserving jars, specimen jars. There were surgical and gynaecological implements, repeated, repeated. Saws and vices, forceps and tweezers, stethoscopes, breast-pumps and urinary bottles. Shelves of artificial nipples, lead and silver, rubber and bakelite. Prostheses of all kinds, noses, ears, breasts, penises, wooden hands, mechanical hands, wire feet, booted feet, artificial buttocks, endless faded hair, in coils, in tangles, in envelopes with the names of the dead men and women from whom it had been clipped.

For the modern visitor, much of the poignancy of Wellcome's collection lies in what we know to be the wrongheadedness of many of the treatments represented by the objects. There are bloodletting bowls, bottles of holy water, amulets to cure bronchitis and Goa stones – made from a paste of clay, crushed shell, amber, musk and resin, and used as antidotes to poisons. Many of them, of course, offered the best odds in a medical science which was full of uncertainty; examining the objects, it is impossible not to feel grateful that we live in a world in which, despite the continuing drawbacks of medicine, many of the diseases and complaints that could spell personal tragedy in the past are treatable as a matter of routine. We have often reflected, too, that, thanks to the mapping of the human genome and the infant science of biotechnology, the medicine of the 21st century will before long seem as outmoded as many of the techniques reflected in Wellcome's things.

'Body Art', however, explores a different aspect of medicine, the capacity of individual doctors to harm and heal. The Hippocratic oath notwithstanding, terrible things have been done in the name of medicine, which may not always have the capacity to set things right. 'Body Art' traces the story of a doctor, Damian, and a young artist, Daisy, and their entanglement, professional and personal. Their path to comfort, healing and transformation lies entirely outside medicine – in art, or in nature itself.

Stacked high upon open shelves, laid out in perspex drawers or carefully wrapped in tissue paper and tucked into boxes, each object in Wellcome's collection has been given an accession number which is both painted on the object (in the smallest of scripts) and written on a slip of card which sits alongside it. This number is the key to accessing all of the recorded information about the object. But its story does not end there. Hari Kunzru's series of evocations, 'The Collected', explores the space between the things' existence as museum objects – only the most recent phase of their rich and varied careers – and their former lives: their spirits. Hari's photographs record their current surroundings – the echoing corridors, the acquisition numbers, the filing cabinets – while his words give voice to the phantom presences that haunt the collection: a shrunken head, a memorial locket enclosing a lock of hair, a fragment of tattooed skin.

It had not, at the outset, been our intention to include non-fiction in this book of imaginative responses to Wellcome's things. But as we pondered what we can know about the past, and the nature of the stories we tell ourselves about what has gone before, it began to seem unreasonable to draw too strict a line between fiction and non-fiction. Our fiction writers, as we know from our extensive exchanges, were priming their imaginations with a thorough grounding in the known facts about their chosen objects – although very often that knowledge was incomplete, or suffused with an unnerving air of off-the-cuff extemporisation. There seemed to be room for a different approach to Wellcome's objects: to take a discrete group of them, look at the evidence, and simply see where the 'facts' might lead. To our delight, in 'Phantom Limbs *or* The Case of Captain Aubert and the Bengal Tiger', Gaby Wood chose to look at the poignant world of prostheses – we, too, had often paused in the Orthopaedics room, with its stack of well-worn arms, legs and crutches, and its distinctive bodily smell, wondering what stories of loss and, we hoped, degrees of recovery might lie behind each of the objects. Gaby's investigation, we feel, combines the strictest historical rigour – in its definition as closeness to the known sources – with the highest degree of sympathetic imagination; and her path leads us straight back to one of the oldest forms of storytelling, the fairytale. Storytelling, after all, is not always about making things up; and some of the best stories are true.

Among the most distant objects in Wellcome's collection, in terms of time, modern medical practice and the ways we now think about our bodies, are the votive offerings. Eyes, hands, breasts, ears, penises and even uteruses, roughly shaped from clay, these were physical lookalikes made to plead with, propitiate or thank the gods that govern the world in sickness and in health. Some of the oldest examples represented in the collection date as far back as the fourth century BC. Their inclusion, in huge numbers, in the collection demonstrates not only Wellcome's determination to chart the science of medicine from its humble beginnings, but also his sympathy with pre-scientific ideas about the body. As a character in Tobias Hill's story – to jump ahead a little – advises one of Wellcome's agents, 'You must buy many things for this history of medicine. Not only medicines. You must buy all the things that people put their belief in.' Helen Cleary has written about a Roman terracotta offering; 'In The Venus Time of Year' juxtaposes a contemporary story with one from the time of the making of her chosen object. Even in a world characterised by flux, some things stay the same: the significance of her object, it turns out, remains unchanged.

From the beginning, we wanted to include the objects themselves – or, to respect the limitations of books, visual representations of them – rather than only words about them. That is why this is an illustrated book, and why the illustrations and the text are so closely entwined. It is also why we wanted to include a graphic short story. In commissioning Peter Blegvad, whose 'Leviathan' series we had long admired, we were also unknowingly harnessing an obsession, as deep as Henry Wellcome's was wide: Peter's contribution, on the subject of milk, draws on a lifetime's reluctant preoccupation with the subject. His method was simply to type 'milk' into the search engines of the Wellcome Library and the Science Museum, and see what happened. The results were dramatic: 'The ground shook, the earth swelled, a geyser gushed forth of matters lactic!' His tour of an imaginary exhibition on the subject of milk, drawn from Wellcome's things, is undertaken in the hope that it will prove purgative: 'I want to be weaned!'

Something that is apt to make any visit to the Wellcome objects in Blythe House a melancholy experience is the consciousness that everything here – including the building itself – is gradually falling into a state of decay. There is, however, a striking exception: a nineteenth-century inductor coil that oozes a hard, honey-coloured slime. In its setting – surrounded by some rather Heath-Robinsonish electrotherapeutic devices – it is so extraordinary as to seem mysteriously, unsettlingly alive. Tobias Hill tells a story about the journey in 1928 on which Peter Johnston Johnston-Saint – one of Wellcome's most faithful agents – acquired the piece.

*

Given the stubborn, uncommunicative permanence of Wellcome's things, their inscription into beliefs about the body and the world that are now irrecoverably past, their undoubted roles in stories of human suffering, it might have been supposed that the responses we commissioned would have been of a sombre cast. The results, as things have turned out, have been quite the reverse. Rather than a reminder of human suffering and the fact that we, too, must die, this book is full of subtle resolutions, quiet shifts toward the light. We offer it, not as a memento mori, but rather as a monumentum vitae – a memorial to the millions of lives that the objects in the Wellcome's collection have touched (patients, doctors, apothecaries, makers, hawkers...) – with an apology for having taken the liberty of having imagined some of them. We have known all along, after all, that we too must die; what is, as far as we know, far more interesting – where the common ground lies – is that we too are alive. Memento mori, as Latin scholars remind us, has become a noun in English; but it is, of course, really a verbal phrase meaning 'remember to die' or 'remember that you will die'. And so we also proffer, as a motto for this book, the reverse sentiment: memento vivere – remember that you are alive!

Lastly, some thanks. Sharp-eyed readers will note that something that has made its way into more than one of the stories is the figure of a baby – wished-for in Helen Cleary's story, new-born in A. S. Byatt's, and voracious in Peter Blegvad's. These presences perhaps owe something to a hitherto unacknowledged collaborator on this project, Hildi's daughter Sophia, who spent many long and exceptionally good-natured afternoons of her babyhood in the corridors of the Blythe House store. Thank you, Sophia.

Our thanks also to Paul Forty at Profile Books and Simon Elliott at Rose Design, both of whom have shown a special empathy with our larger aim: to define a new genre of books exploring the lives that objects have touched by holding them to our ears and seeing what we can hear.

Hildi Hawkins
Danielle Olsen

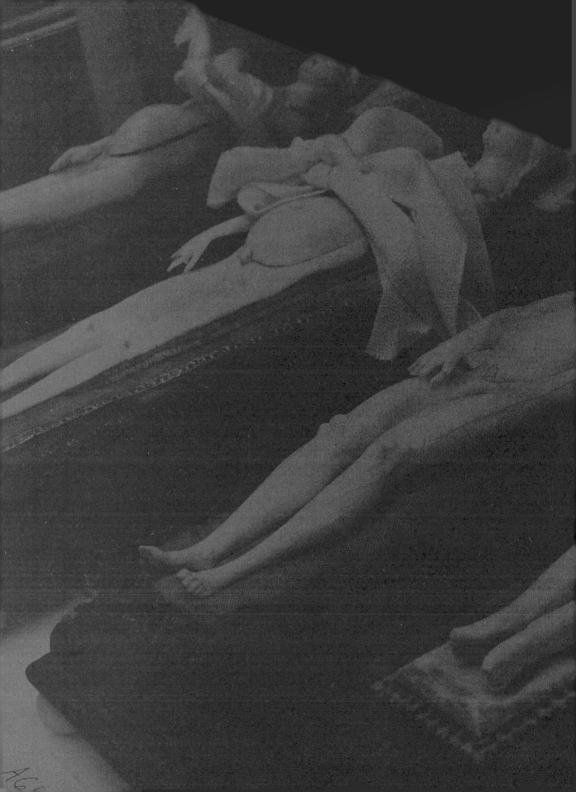

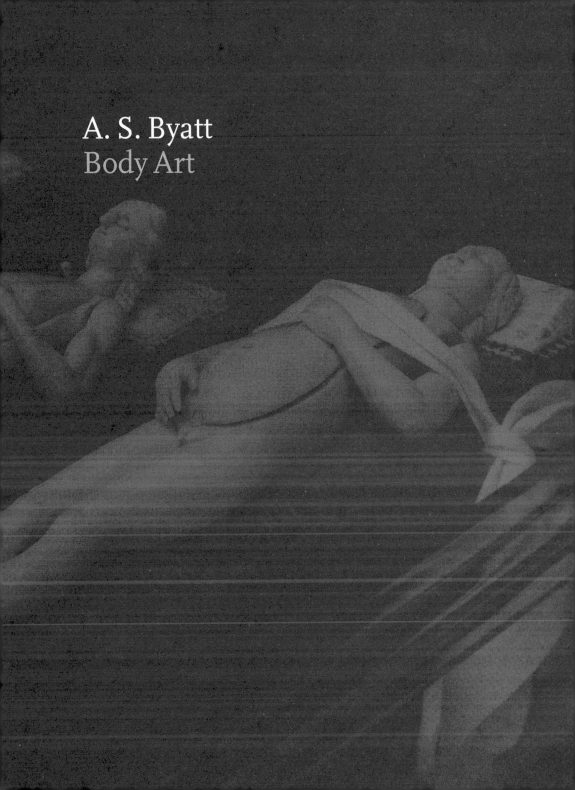

A. S. Byatt
Body Art

Tab. 1.

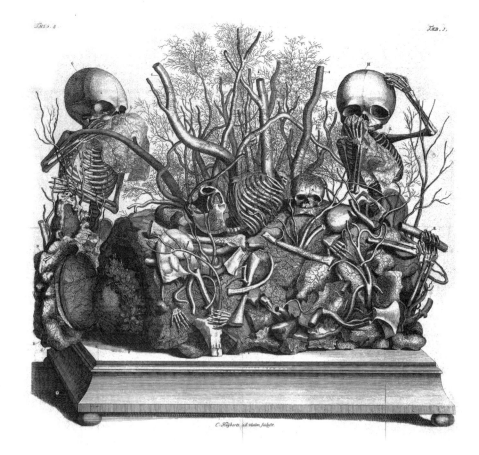

C. Huyberts. ad vivum sculpsit.

THERE WAS CUSTOMARY BANTER in the Gynae Ward at St Pantaleon's, about the race to bear the Christmas Day baby. Damian Becket, making his round after a sleepless night of blood and danger, didn't join in. His newest patient was at the furthest end of the cavernous ward, in the curtained-off section reserved for those who had lost, or might lose, their babies, and those whose babies were damaged or threatened. Dr Becket frowned a little as he strode between the beds, not quite hearing the mewing and gulping of the infants or the greetings of the women. He was frowning, partly because his patient's new baby, a scrap of skin and bone in an incubator in Intensive Care, was not doing well. He was also frowning because he was so tired that he couldn't remember his patient's name. He did not like to admit a fault. The baby should be doing better. His brain should respond to his need to identify people.

He did not notice the stepladder until he had almost crashed into it. It was very tall, made of very shiny aluminium, and was directly under a circular fluorescent light fitting. He stopped suddenly, didn't swear, felt sick because his reactions were slow, and stared upwards into the light, which blinded him. At the top of the ladder, perched precariously on tiptoe, was a figure in what seemed to be a haze of pale filmy garments. Its head was a ball of shiny white spikes. Dr Beckett said that the ladder was dangerous, and should be got out of the way. From the hands of the creature on top of it fluttered scarlet streamers, which glittered wetly in the too-much light. It emitted a ghostly tinkling. *What is going on*, asked Dr Becket, staring grimly upwards.

The Staff Nurse said it was his idea, Dr Becket's idea. It was one of the art students, said Nurse McKitterick, who had given up time and materials to cheer the place up in an original way. Dr Becket had suggested it to the

Art-School Liaison Committee, such a clever idea...Yes, yes, yes, said Dr
Becket, I see. It looks a little dangerous. His tired senses took in the fact
that the ward beyond the ladder was crisscrossed with a rainbow of
coloured strips of plastic, and strips of Indian-looking cloth spangled with
mirror-glass. There were also brass bells and clusters of those eye-shaped
beads that ward off the Evil Eye. They did lighten the darkness of the upper
vaulting. They also emphasised it.

His patient, whose name, Yasmin Muller, was of course written on the
end of her bed, was sobbing quietly. She looked guilty when she opened
her swollen eyelids and saw Dr Becket's severe young face staring down at
her. She said she was sorry, and he said he didn't see what she had to be
sorry about. His fingers were gentle. He said she was rather a mess but it
couldn't be helped and would improve. She asked after her son. Dr Becket
said he was hanging in. He was strong, in so far as anyone born so much
too soon could be strong. It is early days, said Dr Becket, who had
concluded that exact truthfulness was almost always the best path to take,
though the quantity of truth might vary. We can't tell yet what will happen,
he said gravely, reasonably, sensibly. She saw him in a blur, for the first
time really. A wiry man in his early forties, with a close-cut cap of soft dark
hair, slightly bloodshot eyes and a white coat. She said, out of her own
drugged drowsiness, 'You look as though you should get some rest.' And
he frowned again, for he did not like personal remarks, and he particularly
did not like to appear to be in need of anything.

On his way back he remembered the ladder, and was about to sidestep,
when the whole rickety structure began to sway and then toppled. Damian
Becket put out a steady hand, directed the thing itself away from the bed it
threatened, and staggered back under the full weight of the falling artist,
whose head hit his chest, whose skinny ankles were briefly flung over his
shoulder. He clutched; his arms were full of light, light female flesh and
bone, wound up in the rayon and muslin harem trousers and tunic,
embroidered in gold and silver. His nose was in baby-soft, silver-dyed,
spun-glass spikes of hair. Lumpy things began to bounce on the floor.
Bitten apples, a banana, a bent box of chocolates. The woman in the

nearest bed laid claim, loudly, to these last. '*That's* where my chocolates went, I was looking all over, there was only a few left, I was blaming the cleaners.' The person in Dr Becket's arms had quite definitely lost consciousness. Her skin was cold and clammy; her breathing was irregular. There was not, of course, a spare bed to put her on, so he carried her along the ward, and out into the nurses' area, followed by his entourage. There he laid her carefully across the desk, felt her pulse, flicked up her eyelids. She seemed bloodless and anaemic. Skinny.

'Just a simple faint,' he said, as she opened her eyes and took him in. 'In need of a good meal, I'd say, whatever else.'

She had a nice little pointed face, rendered grotesque, in his view, by gold studs and rings in pierced lips and nostrils. She was white like milled flour. She sat up and pulled her shapeless garments around her. 'I'm so sorry,' she said in a breathy voice. 'I'm OK now. I hope nothing got broken.'

'Mr Becket saved the situation,' said the Staff Nurse. 'Did you slip?'

'I felt dizzy. I don't like heights.'

'What were you doing up there in those impractical clothes, in that case?' asked Damian.

'It was a nice idea. To decorate the ward. I offered.'

She sat, slightly hunched, on the edge of the desk, swinging white-stockinged feet in streamlined modern nubuck clogs, with high wedged soles, open at the back. They were a dull crimson, stained with splashes of paint, or glue. Damian Becket bit back a remark about the idiocy of climbing ladders in such footwear, and asked instead

'When did you last eat?'

'I don't really remember. I was late for here, so I just ran out.'

'I was going to take myself to the canteen for brunch. Would you like to join me?'

The nurses had piled the pocketed fruit on the desk beside her. She did not look at it.

'OK,' she said. 'If you like.'

*

They went down to the basement canteen in a service lift, accompanied by two green-gowned theatre porters and a trolley. The artist shivered, possibly because she was cold, which she should have been, in those clothes. He said

'I'm Damian Becket. And you?'

'I'm Daisy. Daisy Whimple.'

They went into the canteen, which had moulded imitation wood plastic chairs, circa 1960, and some unexpected prints, bright abstracts full of movement, on pale green walls. There was the usual smell of cooking fat, and a clatter of steel teapots. She hesitated in the doorway, and her white face grew whiter. He told her she didn't look too good, found her a seat, and asked what he could bring her.

'Whatever. Well, preferably vegetables. I try to be a vegan.'

He came back with an English breakfast for himself and a vegetarian pasta dish for her, with a tomato side salad. The pasta was pinkish and grey-green corkscrews, covered with some kind of cheese sauce. She ate the tomato, and turned the fusilli over and over with her fork, in the aimless way of children trying to heap leftovers to make them look smaller. Damian Becket, having eaten two sausages, two rashers of bacon, a fried egg, a heap of fried potatoes and a spoonful of baked beans, felt more human and studied Daisy Whimple more carefully. Anaemic almost certainly, anorexic possibly. An odd limpness in the wrists. He couldn't really see her body in the furls of her clothing but he had held it in his arms, and it was young and tautly constructed. She had blue eyes and sky-blue painted lashes. The veins in her thin arms were also very blue, as was a kind of traced tattoo like lacy flowers, that infested her lower arms like the evening mittens of Edwardian ladies. Her nails had been very neatly bitten.

'You should eat *something*. If you don't eat meat and things, you know, you in fact need to eat *more*, to keep up the protein.'

'I'm sorry. It's nice of you. I feel sick, that's really the problem, with the ladder and all that.'

He asked her about herself. He was not good at this. He was a good doctor, but he had no skill at talking, no ease of manner, he didn't in fact want to know the details of other human lives, except in so far as he needed to know facts and histories in order to save those lives. He was unaware that his conventional good looks were to a certain extent a substitute for amiability. Even now, he was thinking, if she talked a bit, she might lose her nervous tension and be able to be hungry. He imagined her from inside her body. Her cramped little stomach.

She said she was a student at the Spice Merchants' School of Art. She had wanted to be a designer – well, it was all she had ever been any good at at school, her education had been – with a fleeting look up at his face – much interrupted, rather haphazard. But really she wanted to be an artist. She had taken part in one or two joint studio shows, with the people she worked with. Some people quite liked her stuff. Her voice trailed away. She said she'd seen the notice in the art school asking for volunteers to make things for the wards, and she thought it was a really nice idea. So she'd come. She was surprised there weren't more. More students there, that was.

'Please try to eat something. Would you prefer anything else – fruit, a roll and butter, some cake – '

'Everything seems to turn my stomach. I'll eat when I get back.'

He asked where she lived.

'Oh well, like, I sleep on my boyfriend's studio floor. Lots of us do that. There's lots of studio space in the old warehouses. Once they get done up of course they go for astronomic prices, the floor space, but people like students and such get like temporary bases in the ones that aren't done up – or not done up yet – you can get nasty surprises, your feet go through the floors and that kind of thing. But it's OK, it's a roof, and a workspace.'

She said, doubtfully, she'd better be going then. She was still forking over the fusilli. He remarked that they were nasty colours, unappetising really, fleshy and mouldy. This interested her. She reconsidered the pasta. You're right, she told him, it's meant to look appetising, tomato juice, spinach. It looks a bit disgusting. Dead, maybe. Lots of colours are sort of deathly. You have to be careful. He said he liked the brightness of her decorations. They were in keeping with the hospital's modern art collection. Had she seen that? She said she had seen some of it, and meant to get a look at the rest while she was on this project. She stood up to go. She looked as pale as ever, no hint of any kind of pink, either deathly or flushed with energy. He said he would walk her to the door. She said he didn't have to, she was fine. He said he was going home anyway.

They stopped in the new entrance lobby round the central stairwell. Stainless steel and glass doors and cubicles had been fitted incongruously into the late-Victorian red brick. The brick was that very hot, peppery red of the Victorian Gothic. The brick walls were decorated with panels of encaustic tiles, depicting chillies and peppercorns, vanilla pods and tea leaves, nutmegs and cloves. St Pantaleon's stood in Pettifer Street, just where it joined Whittington Passage. It was in Wapping, not so far from Wapping Old Stairs. It had once been a workhouse, which had become the Spice Merchants' Lying-in Hospital, to which was attached the Molly Pettifer Clinic for the Treatment of the Diseases of Women. It had become St Pantaleon's when the new National Health Service refurbished it in 1948, adding prefabricated temporary buildings which still stood. Sir Eli Pettifer had been a surgeon who had worked with the East India Company and with the British Army in India and in other places. He had written a treatise on the medical uses of culinary spices, and had made a fortune, through judicious speculation in spice cargoes. His daughter, Molly, had been one of the first generation of qualified women doctors, many of whom were allowed to train because a need was perceived for their ministrations in the Empire. Like many of them, Molly had been carried away by typhoid, whilst practising obstetrics and general surgery in Calcutta. Pettifer had endowed the hospital for her, and persuaded the Spice Merchants to endow it more richly still. He had left it his huge Collection, mostly of medical instruments and curiosities, with the injunction that it be made available for the instruction and amazement of the general public. It occupied several locked strong-rooms in the basement, whilst much of it was still crated, and much more heaped haphazardly in dusty display cabinets.

One of the paintings from the Collection, a Dutch painting of an anatomy lesson being performed on a stillborn infant, had hung in the entrance hall. It had been Damian Becket's idea to take it down and put it in the Hospital Committee Room, replacing it with a large abstract print by Albert Irvin, which Damian himself had donated. Carried away by the brilliance of Irvin's powerful brushstrokes, pink and gold, scarlet and royal blue, woven with emerald and flicks of white, he had talked the hospital into collecting other modern works, inviting sponsors, talking the artists into loans and concessions. Painted banners by Noel Forster floated down from the inside of the Gothic tower. Huge abstract visions of almost-vases and possible-seashores by Alan Gouk, in bristly slicks of paint – purple, sulphur, puce, lime – ran along the walls. In the corridors were Herons and Terry Frosts, Hodgkins and Hoylands. A Paolozzi machine-man glittered, larger than life, next to the reception pigeonhole. There was an Art Committee, who usually followed Damian's suggestions. They had also put him in charge of the Pettifer Collection, which he knew he should look at, go into, catalogue, arrange, only he was so tired, and there was so little money, and so many sick women, and he preferred his abstract modernist brightness. Indeed, 'preferred' was too weak a word.

So he was a little put out when Daisy Whimple stared dutifully up at the banners, cast her eye over the brushstrokes and said unenthusiastically 'Yeah, very nice, very colourful. Pretty.'

'What sort of work do you do?' asked Damian Becket levelly. 'Not like this, I take it.'

'Well, no, not like this at all. I'm into installations, or I would be if there was any space anywhere I could get to install anything.'

'The things you are doing in the ward are – are bright.'

'Yeah, I figured that was what was wanted. I mean, like, the notice actually used the words *cheer up* the wards, didn't it? I agree, really, you want easy cheerful art when you're in one of those places. Easy on the eye, yes. For *Christmas* and all that.'

'But you haven't – installed – anything to do with Christmas. No snow, no Christmas tree, no reindeers. No crèche.'

'No one asked for a crèche. I can't do that sort of stuff. It's all *kitsch*.'

There was venom in the word. She added

'And I don't suppose the establishment'd be too happy if I like, *sent it up*, the angels and stars and stuff. Though the angels are the bit I don't mind.'

He asked, on an impulse, which modern artists she really admired. The answer came quick, without time taken for reflection, as though it were part of a credo.

'Beuys. He was the greatest. He changed everything.'

He was piqued to find that not much came into his mind, à propos of Beuys. He dredged.

'Didn't he work in fat and felt?'

She looked at him kindly. 'Among other things. He worked with himself too. He sat for days and months on a stage with a coyote.'

Damian said foolishly that you could hardly have a coyote in a hospital.

'I know that. I'm doing what was expected OK, OK?'

'OK.'

He said that he would be very interested to see her work when she had finished it. He said he hoped she would get a proper meal. He said he was going to get a taxi home, and could he drop her anywhere. She said no, she needed fresh air. Thanks.

They parted. It was cold outside: an icy wind was blowing in off the Thames. It fluttered in her silly clothes, and ruffled her silver hair. He resisted an impulse to run after her and lend her his overcoat.

He lived in a Dockland apartment, glass-walled and very modern, looking over at Canary Wharf. It was simultaneously austere and brilliant. His furniture was chrome and glass and black leather. His carpet was iron grey. His walls were white, and were hung with abstract works – several of Patrick Heron's 1970s silkscreens, some of Noel Forster's intricately interlaced ribbons of colour, resembling rose windows, a Hockney print of cylinders, cones and cubes, a framed poster of Matisse's *Snail*. He had also one or two brilliant Korean silk cushions in traditional green, gold, shocking pink and blue. He lived alone, since his parting from his wife, with whom he did not communicate. He considered himself hopelessly and helplessly married. He was a lapsed Catholic – this was something about himself that rose to the surface whenever –

which was rarely – he was in a position where he was required to give a personal description of himself. He could have added adverbs – savagely lapsed, insistently lapsed, even in some sense devoutly lapsed. His way of life – including his attitude to his marriage – still ran furiously along the narrow channels cut by his upbringing.

His Northern Irish mother had meant him for the priesthood. He was to be her gift to God, she often said, having also decided that his elder brothers were to be teacher and republican politician, which they now were, showing, perhaps, the power of her gentle certainties. His father was himself a schoolteacher, specialising in Irish Literature, and had wanted Damian to be what he himself had not been, a true scholar, a linguist who spoke many tongues, a civilised man. Damian had tried to please both of them. They were kind and their tongues were golden. He had got as far as reading literature at University College Dublin, where he met his wife, Eleanor, who meant to be an actress, who had become since they parted a successful actress on the television. Eleanor was a good girl, and was tormented – in those distant days – by problems about contraception. She tormented Damian in turn, leaving him both overexcited and perpetually unsatisfied. They married, as a direct consequence, when she was 18 and he was 19. Eleanor's sister Rosalie was 17, not scholarly, and not a good girl. She once got drunk at a party, at the height of Damian's time of overexcited frustration, and had suddenly stripped off her jumper and bra in a boxroom where they were hunting for coats. She stood and stared at him, wild-eyed, wild-haired, laughing, and the great brown eyes of her large freckled breasts seemed to stare at him too. She told him not to be in a hurry. She told him her sister was a cold little fish, he hadn't the wit to see it because he didn't know enough women. He took her jumper and bra and made her put them back on. She went on laughing. A year later she was dead; she bled to death after a back-street abortion. In his dreams he still saw the spheres of her breasts, and the constellation of freckles, and the blind puckered brown eyes of her nipples.

*

He did not lose his faith as a consequence of her death. Nor as a consequence of its effect on Eleanor, who now wriggled away from his body as though he was going to damage or contaminate her. Nor out of any moral outrage – though he felt some – at the Church's interference in processes he wanted to believe were human and natural. (That included contraception. Human beings were not animals. They cared for children for perhaps a third of the normal human life. They needed to have the number of children they could decently and responsibly care for. Their sexual desires were unfortunately not periodic in the way of cows and bitches. Women were perpetually on heat unless, as in the case of his wife, the heat had been turned off. It followed that contraception was natural.) He lost his faith as a result of a vision.

The vision was conventional enough, in one sense. It was a vision of Christ on the Cross – not a heavenly appearance, but the result of an unnaturally close inspection of the carving that hung in his local church, a painted wooden carving, neither good nor bad, a mediocre *run-of-the-mill* carving of a human body, unpleasantly suspended from nails hammered through the palms of hands neither writhing in pain nor distorted by stress, but spread wide in blessing. He thought, the anatomy is bad, the weight would rip through muscle and sinew long before the man was dead. Some crucifixes did support the feet. This one did not. They were crossed, and improbably nailed through both ankles. Some care had been taken to depict the agony of the muscles of the torso, the arms and the thighs. The gash under the heart had realistic slipperiness where it opened; unreal immobilised paint-blood spilled from it, in runnels someone had taken pleasure in varying. There were no bloodstains on the loincloth, which carefully obscured the sex. The face was stylised. Long, unlined, with downcast eyelids, closed as in sleep, and a mouth slightly opened, showing no teeth. More artistic blood had been dribbled from the clutches of the crown of thorns in the abundant shaggy hair. The dead or dying flesh – the carving *was simply not good enough for him to be sure which* – was creamy in colour, with pink highlights. He thought, I belong to a religion which worships the form of a dead or dying man. He realised that he did not believe and never had believed either that the man's bodily death had been reversed or that he ascended into heaven, for there was no heaven, and all human descriptions of heaven made it pathetically clear that we can't imagine it well enough to make it at all attractive as a prospect. He would not meet poor Rosalie in any such place, and he did not think he would even want to. He did not believe that this one unpleasant death had in any way cancelled out the sins of the earth: Rosalie's wildness, the Church's obstructiveness and bloodymindedness, his grandfathers' deaths in bomb blasts in wartime (paternal) and peacetime (maternal). He *never had believed* any of it. He felt for the shape of the time – his whole life – when he would have said he believed, and was aghast to sense it like a great humming ice-box behind him, in which what he had been had kept its form, neither dead nor alive, suspended. He was a human bowed down under the weight of a man-sized ice-box.

He went on looking at the figure hanging by his hands, with outrage and then with pity. There was a man, who had been dying, and then dead. And there was an idea of who he was, which was a dream, which was a poem, which was a moral cage, which was a film over a clear vision of things. A man is his body, his body is a man.

From which it followed that Damian Becket, having straightened his back, and shaken the ice-box from his shoulders to melt, he hoped, at the feet of the lifeless carving, had to concern himself with bodies. His vision had not taught him that everything was without meaning, that chaos reigned. There was order, but order was in time and space and the body. If a man – who had seen the ice-box – wanted to make sense of his life and live well, he must concern himself with the body. There were multifarious reasons why in his case it was the female body. His decision to become a medical student, at the age when he should have been about to earn his living, offended his mother and made his wife extremely angry. He was not quite sure why she was so very angry, and could not find out. Communication is much harder in intimate fear and anger than between casual companions. Silence spread into their lives.

He went to London and she did not. She went to church, and he did not.

He discovered colour, at the same time as he took up the post at St Pantaleon's. Every time he came home, he stared at the bright forms on his walls, and worshipped the absence of God in the material staining of paint and ink.

He saw Daisy Whimple several more times during his visits to the Gynae Wards in the days before Christmas. She seemed to be the only student who had chosen to work on that ward – the take-up of the hospital offer had indeed been rather disappointing. She had made several bouquets or bundles of odd things suspended from the ceiling – children's whirligigs, coloured feathers, plastic bubble-wrapping stitched with cut-up plastic beakers and bottles, green and blue. He could see her sitting cross-legged on the floor in the corner of the ward, wound in a coil of tape to which she was stitching plumage – hen-feathers, turkey-feathers, black feathers which shone like oil. He stopped once and asked her how all this was funded. She said oh, she had scrounged most of it. She said, if you look closely at a lot of these things – the little whirlies, the gauze flowers – you'll see that they're rejects, a bit torn. They look fine like this, if you don't examine them too closely. He said he would see she got reimbursed, all the same.

'I like doing it,' she said. 'It's my pleasure.'

She said 'I'm putting the really colourful bits at the miserable end.'

'The miserable end?'

'The no-hopers. The dead babies and tied-up-tubes end. Sodding rotten luck to have to lie there and listen to other people's kids squealing all night and not getting any sleep. I think you lot are cruel, if you want to know.'

He said 'Beds are in short supply.'

She said, with a return of the sudden venom that cut through her pale daffiness,

'I know all about that. All about that. The consultants are overworked, they have to have all their cases next to each other to get round, bad wombs next to good wombs and no-wombs mixed in. I do know about that.'

'I'm sorry,' he said. He wasn't a man for arguing. He walked onwards.

The Sister said 'She was in here last year, you know. Abortion with complications. Mr Cuthbertson operated.'

Mr Cuthbertson had subsequently left, after several of his patients had been discovered to have been badly handled. Damian looked a question at the Sister.

'Raging infection of the tubes. Lost an ovary.'

He did not want to appear to be prying, so dropped the question. He could look it up in the records. But there was no need for him to know the gynaecological history of Daisy Whimple, who was trailing paper garlands of sunflowers and pheasant feathers between the bed-heads of the no-hopers.

The Christmas baby was black twins, huge, healthy, and slow to deliver. Damian was there because there were complications, and because he liked to work on holy days and holidays. The ward, when they wheeled their patient in, was largely empty. The mothers and the no-mothers had Christmas cards on their lockers. Daisy Whimple's decorations spun and fluttered in the draught from the double doors. Daisy Whimple was sitting at the Sister's desk, eating a pot of strawberry yogurt. Damian said

'I'm surprised to see you. You've made it all look lovely. But I thought you'd have gone home for the holiday, by now.'

'Home?' said Daisy. 'No, I haven't gone home.' She looked at him rather bleakly. 'You haven't gone home, either.'

'I was needed – '

'I've made myself useful in a small way,' said Daisy, looking at the Staff Nurse for confirmation. 'Haven't I?'

'You've been great.'

'I wasn't criticising. I was just asking.'

He waited for her to say, 'Well, you've asked, now sod off.' But she just bent her fragile neck over the yogurt, and ended the conversation.

He asked the Staff Nurse, when Daisy had left, what she thought Daisy lived on. Did she have a grant, or what? The Staff Nurse said she didn't know. She did seem to be coming in to get warm. 'She hugs the radiators, when I'm not looking,' said Nurse Ogunbiyi. 'And she nicks things off the lockers and the trays going back to the kitchen. I gave her that yogurt. She talks nice enough, tells you little things, but she don't say where she lives at present, nor yet if she's got any cash.'

Once or twice, when the Christmas holidays were over, he thought he saw her flitting round the corners of corridors, or stepping into the lift. But he couldn't be sure. And he was tired, and she wasn't his business, his business was flesh, and its making, mending, and unmaking.

On Twelfth Night the decorations were taken down by the hospital cleaners.

He thought of Daisy Whimple again when the Hospital Art Collection Committee met in the boardroom, under Sir Eli Pettifer's Dutch painting of the anatomy lesson. There stood the doctor, stretching out the taut umbilical cord in two fastidious fingers. There lay the dead child, its belly opened like a flower, still attached to the veined medusa-like mound, which had been part of its mother. There stood the black-robed Dutchmen, looking solemnly at the painter. There, oddly, was a small boy, aged perhaps ten, also black-robed, holding up the skeleton of a child of roughly the same size as the peaceful corpse under dissection. The skull smiled; skulls always do; it was the only smile in the serious painting. Martha Sharpin, who was early for the meeting, like Damian, said to him that it was historically interesting as to whether the skeletal child was a religious *memento mori* or simply an anatomical demonstration. She believed it must be religious, because of the odd age of the child who held it up. Damian said that as a lapsed Catholic he wanted to believe it was simply an elegant way of presenting anatomical facts. He had a horror, he said, of the musty world of relics and bits of skin and bone which ought no longer to have meaning if their ex-inhabitants were in heaven. Martha Sharpin said he was forgetting the resurrection of the body, for one thing. And for another, the stillborn were not in heaven but in limbo, forever unbaptised.

'Are you a Catholic?'

'No,' said Martha Sharpin, 'an art historian'.

Martha represented the Spice Merchants' Foundation on the Committee. She was the Foundation's Arts Co-ordinator, new to the job, having succeeded Letitia Holm, an elderly aesthete from the second generation of Bloomsbury. She was regarded, with approval, as 'new blood' by the distinguished trustees of the Foundation, and also with suspicion, as very young, and possibly lacking gravitas. She had a Courtauld PhD – her subject had been the Vanitas in seventeenth-century painting – and a subsequent qualification in Arts Administration. She was in her thirties, with smooth, dark, well-cut hair and a strong-featured bony face. Her skin was golden, possibly with a hint of the oriental. She had very black brows and lashes, and dark chocolate-brown eyes: she appeared to wear no make-up, and appeared to need none. She wore the usual well-cut black trouser suit, and a scarf made of some shimmering, permanently pleated textile in silver-blue, pinned, with a large glass mosaic brooch, into a shape that resembled the stocks and neckties of the people in the painting. Damian Becket liked the look of her. This was the second time they had met, the second Committee meeting they had both attended. She had decided he was the mover and shaker of this committee, and that she needed to get to know him. She said

'I have to say, the installation in the entrance hall is marvellous. Makes you want to sing, which is hard, in a hospital. Letitia told me you were the one with the ideas.'

'Letitia was very helpful to me about where to buy things for myself. I buy prints. My very first was a print by Bert Irvin called Magdalen. We bought one for the second floor, too. Rushing coloured forms, with grey. I puzzled about why it was called Magdalen – being a lapsed Catholic. Irvin names his work quite arbitrarily for the roads round his studio. I like that. Grey road, rushing colours.'

'You collect?'

'I wouldn't call it that. I buy prints. Tell me about Joseph Beuys.'

The connection seemed odd to Martha, who raised her thick brows and opened her mouth, just as the rest of the Committee came in. An almoner, a nursing supervisor, the Bursar, a representative from the Art College, a junior lawyer from the Spice Merchants. The Art College representative was a performance artist whose attendance and attention at the meetings were both erratic. When he spoke, which was very infrequently, he spoke in sentences like unravelling knitting, with endless dependent clauses depending on dependent clauses ending in lacunae and stuttering. Letitia Holm had disliked and despised him. She said his conversation was like his art, which consisted of a kind of hopeless-Houdini self-suspension from anything upright – lampposts, railway bridges, river bridges – in cradles or bags of knotted ropes of all thicknesses. Damian did not know what Martha Sharpin thought of him. He needed to find out.

The meeting wound on. Damian reported the purchase of a painting by Therese Oulton and the gift by an anonymous donor of some prints by Tom Phillips. The nursing supervisor reported on the scheme for ward decoration by the art students. She said there had been problems with someone trying to bring unhygienic things into the ward with the incubators. And some of the students had started things and not come back, leaving bits of mistletoe and oranges with cloves, cluttering the surgical ward. Damian Becket said he thought the decoration of the Gynae Ward had been very successful, very imaginative and unusual. He thought they should thank Miss Whimple. He asked Joey Blount, the performance artist, if he knew Miss Whimple. Not personally, said Joey Blount. Not at all, actually.

The meeting always ended with the problem of Eli Pettifer's Collection, which was always deferred. It was a condition of the bequest – and of all Pettifer's other munificent bequests – that the Collection should be maintained and appropriately displayed. And there it was, in boxes, and old display cabinets you couldn't make your way between. Daunting. They'd once had a real cataloguer, said the Bursar, who had been in there for six months, and got very depressed by the dust and the darkness. She turned out to have catalogued *one box* when she left, according to a system no one could make head or tail of. Moreover, she'd developed a mystery virus, which she claimed must have come out of the boxes, and had threatened to sue the hospital.

Martha asked whether the Collection was labelled. Yes, said the Bursar, most of it had little handwritten stickers and tags. It was hard to know where to start, he said gloomily. Martha said she would like to see it. The Bursar said this was more than Letitia had offered to do. Letitia was squeamish. Martha said she herself was not, and would take a look at what was there. Damian said he would be happy to show her round.

So Damian Becket and Martha Sharpin made a clanking descent in the steel cage into the bowels of the hospital. The door to the Collection was opened by a coded keyboard: Damian punched in his code and pushed it open. Martha Sharpin exclaimed at the extent of it. There were several rooms, opening off a central one which had a little murky daylight from a thick glass window let into the pavement above, through which they could see the soles of passing feet. There were rooms within rooms, made of crates and packing cases. There were cabinets along the walls of the rooms containing shelf after shelf of medical implements and curiosities. Martha walked along, staring in. Damian followed her.

Shelf after shelf after shelf of syringes – cartridge syringes, laryngeal syringes, varicose vein syringes, haemorrhoid syringes, lachrymal syringes, exhausting syringes, made from ivory and ebony, brass and steel. From another cabinet shelf after shelf of glass eyes stared at them from neatly segmented boxes, or squinnied higgledy-piggledy, like collections of marbles. There were bottles – ancient tear-bottles, ornate pharmacy bottles in pale rose with gilded letters, preserving jars, specimen jars. There were surgical and gynaecological implements, repeated, repeated. Saws and vices, forceps and tweezers, stethoscopes, breast-pumps and urinary bottles. Shelves of artificial nipples, lead and silver, rubber and bakelite. Prostheses of all kinds – noses, ears, breasts, penises, wooden hands, mechanical hands, wire feet, booted feet, artificial buttocks, and endless faded hair, in coils, in tangles, in envelopes with the names of the dead men and women from whom it had been clipped.

There were specimens also. Human brains and human testicles in jars of formaldehyde. Shelves of foetuses – monkeys, armadillos, rats, sows, boys, girls and an elephant. Monsters also, humans and creatures born with no head, or two heads, stunted arms or spare fingers, conjoined twins and wizened hair-balls. One case, which was arranged with some aesthetic intention, contained a series of nineteenth-century glass ornamental domes – or maybe museum exhibits – in which foetal skeletons were at play with wreaths of dried flowers, wax grapes, skeleton leaves and branches of dead coral. Others contained wax humans divided vertically, fleshed and clothed on the left hand, polished skeleton and skull on the right. Martha lingered over these. She had seen similar things, but never so many, never so strange.

Damian pulled open a tall crate from which wood shavings were emerging. Inside was what looked like a white statue of a goddess, a young woman with closed eyes and a curiously flaccid surface, folds of flesh rolling back towards her spine. He realised that she should be lying on her back, and saw that she was swollen to bursting, a full-term gravid woman. Then he bent to read the label, and saw that what he was seeing was the plaster cast made from the body of one Mercy Parker, who had died on the 24th December 1770. He remembered that such plaster casts were made for teaching purposes. The deliquescent flesh was the other side of rigor mortis.

He closed her in again, and went back to Martha, who was intent on a collection of small ivory women, some occidental, some oriental, each a few inches long, lying in various postures, curved for sleep, or extended. Some of the occidental ones had removable, thimble-sized navel-and-stomach, which could display, and did, the miniature heart, lungs and intestines, or the curled foetus in the womb. Martha asked Damian if they were diagnostic or votive. He said he didn't know. He said, thinking of the lead nipples which must have poisoned what they were intended to purify, that the whole thing was a collection of attempts to preserve and lengthen life, which nevertheless bore witness to human interventions that had drastically shortened it. He pointed at the early gynaecological forceps.

'A huge step forward. But spreading puerperal fever wherever they were used. What am I going to do, Dr Sharpin?'

'Martha, please. You need someone to make a start on conservation advice and cataloguing. Someone brave, who won't get bogged down, and won't be slapdash.'

'Do you know such a paragon?'

'No. But I could work on it – say one afternoon a week – myself, and get it into a state where it could be handed over to a proper curator.'

Damian said he could think of no better solution. Martha said she would be glad if he could provide a dogsbody – someone to lift and dust, and help with labels.

The image of Daisy Whimple, a little inappropriately, visited Damian's mind.

'I know an art student. She did some good decorations in the Gynae Ward, for Christmas.'

'She'd need to be able to spell. It's often not their strong point.'

Damian had no idea whether Daisy could spell. Nor, when he asked in the ward, did any of the nurses know where she lived. Nor when, with unusual persistence for an overworked man, he called the Art College, could they enlighten him, though they promised to speak to her if she came in to classes, which, they said, she mostly didn't. Later, Damian wondered why he hadn't asked them for a competent student who could spell.

Martha Sharpin began her foray at the Collection. She only rarely saw Damian Becket. One day, when they met by pseudo-accident in the lift, she asked if his hours were regular enough for her to take him out for a meal, to talk over a project she had, to put artists-in-residence into hospitals. She thought he was the doctor who might see the point. Damian liked being asked out to dinner by this handsome, sensible woman, who carried her knowledge lightly, and made life more interesting for many people. He found her attractive. He liked looking at women with good clothes, *on* their bodies, so to speak. He saw a lot of female flesh, slippery and sweating, even provocatively pouting and posturing at him. He liked the way Martha's sweaters moved easily around her waist – the sense that she was in control of herself. When they had their dinner, in a dockside restaurant overlooking the rolling grey mist on the Thames, and the snaking lights of the police launches, he admired her trouser suit, wine-coloured this time, fluid and well cut, ornamented with another glass mosaic brooch in the shape of a paisley dangling an absurd pink pearl. He remarked on it. She said it was 'an Andrew Logan. Called Goddess. It has tiny feathers embedded in it, look. Cosmic fertility'.

They enjoyed their dinner. She explained the difficulties of placing artists-in-residence. They had had one once who wanted to photograph breast cancers, blow up the prints, and install them in the patients' waiting area. 'They were spectacular photographs,' she said, 'but inappropriate. Or too *appropriating*. Photography has that quality. They weren't, so to speak, the artist's own cancers to display.'

Damian said he supposed there was no sense placing an abstract colourist in a ward or a waiting-room. Martha asked if he'd found the art student he thought might help with the Collection. What sort of work did she do?

'Well, the decorations were ingenious and colourful. I did get the impression she was so to speak slumming. She said she did installations. She mentioned Beuys.'

'Ah, so that was why you suddenly asked about him – '

'I don't really know about him.'

Martha said he was a great artist who dealt in dark things made of common materials.

'Fat and felt.'

'Exactly. Usually on a large scale. Reliquaries of no religion. Things evoking wars and prison camps. He's probably the greatest single influence on art students today. They do *personal versions* – you know, the fish slice that my girlfriend didn't clean, the knickers I wore when I first kissed Joe Bloggs – the disc collection I pinched from my ex-lover – the purely personal. I am an artist so my relics *are art*. I'm not saying that's your student's line. She may really understand Beuys.'

Damian said he had no idea what she did or didn't understand but he did know she was hungry. Anyway, he couldn't find her. They had better look for another dogsbody. And it didn't sound as though she'd be at all suitable for the placement.

The next day, out of the corner of his eye, he saw the white head and floating clothing whisk round the corner of a corridor. He strode on, making no sign that he had seen anything untoward, and suddenly turned back into the cupboard door she was standing inside.

'Hullo. What are you doing here?'

The small face went through various thought processes without finding a suitable answer.

'I've been trying to find you. I've got a kind of a part-time job I thought might interest you.'

'What kind of a job?' Suspicious, ready to run away.

'Can you spell?'

'As a matter of fact, yes. I was always a good speller. Either you are or you aren't. I am. I always get ten out of ten in those competitions for spelling things like harass and embarrass and sedentary and minuscule, I don't boast of it. It's like being double-jointed.'

'Are you interested in the work?'

'I'm an artist.'

'I know. This is part-time work that would interest an artist.' He wanted to say, a hungry artist, and smile at her, but he stopped himself. He saw her as a hungry child. She saw herself as a woman artist.

Daisy and Martha were installed in the Collection. They put on white hospital overalls and white cotton gloves, and set about the discovery of the treasures and horrors. They worked Friday afternoons. When Damian was not working, he sometimes dropped in to see how they were progressing. All three exclaimed over a bottled foetus wearing bead necklaces around neck, wrists and ankles, or a large cardboard box that proved to contain the wax heads and hands of a group of nineteenth-century murderers, all looking remarkably cheerful. Damian took Martha out to dinner – to return the first invitation, and to discuss the artist-in-residence. They also discussed Daisy, quite naturally, and partly in this context.

Damian asked whether Martha thought Daisy could be the required artist. Martha said Daisy did not discuss her own work, and she, Martha, had no idea what it was like. Daisy was good at the cataloguing work – deft, quick-witted, with a good memory. 'She says funny things about terrible things,' said Martha. 'But I feel she's sad. She says *nothing* personal. I don't know where she lives, or who she hangs out with. She seems to haunt the hospital.'

'I think she scrounges. I think she doesn't get enough to eat. She's got a boyfriend. She says she lives on his studio floor.'

'She intrigues you.'

'She was in the Gynae Ward herself, last year. She had a bad time. I looked her up. It was a bad time that – that the hospital didn't exactly help – '

Martha said every woman must wonder what it felt like to be a man who saw so many women. In extreme situations.

Damian said his profession had made him unnaturally detached. 'I see them as lives and deaths,' he told Martha, 'as problems and dangers, and sometimes as triumphs. Not mostly as people. I'm not good at people'.

Martha smiled at him in the candlelight, and the lights on the river bobbed and swayed. She said

'You're very kind, for a detached man.'

'I'm kind *because* I'm detached. It's no trouble to be kind, if you remember to think of it. And I had a religious upbringing.' He hesitated. He stared at the dark water. He said

'It's odd what persists of a religious upbringing. I've no God and I don't want Him, I don't miss church and all the smells and singing. But I do somehow still consider myself married to my wife, though we haven't seen each other for four or five years now, and hope never to see each other again.'

Martha understood very clearly that she was being offered something. She frowned, and then said

'I've never had a religion, and never been married – never even come close – so I – have to use my imagination. Does your wife consider herself married?'

'She's an actress and a Catholic. That's a daft answer. Do you know, I don't know *what* she thinks.'

One day, looking for Martha, he arrived to find the Collection in darkness and both women away. He began to wander amongst the shelves, when his foot squelched on something. He looked down. It was a potato chip and it was warm. He looked around and saw two more, at intervals. He bent down and touched them. They were both warm. He listened. He could hear his own breathing and what seemed like the sounds of the myriad dead things and outdated artefacts, shifting and settling. But he could hear breath, when he held his own, light breath, breath trying to be silent. He began to search the Collection, listening for a giveaway rustle, and heard nothing, except breath, breath, silence, gasped breath, breath, silence. He stalked quietly, and between a long row of upright packing cases saw another potato chip, and what might be the opening of a burrow. So he peered into the darkness and took out the torch he always carried, and waved the pinpoint of light around in the mouth of the tunnel. Something white trembled vaguely at the other end.

'Don't be frightened,' said Damian kindly. 'Come out.'

Louder breathing, more trembling. Damian went in, and illuminated a nest, made of white cellular blankets, the sort that are on hospital trolleys, old pillows. Daisy sat in the midst of them, oddly clothed in her white coat and gloves. A plastic box of chips nested in the folds of the blankets. Damian said 'If you eat those with those gloves on, you completely destroy the point of the gloves being sterile – well, clean at least – ' Daisy sniffed.

'Are you *living* here?'

'It's temporary. I got kicked out of the studio.'

'When?'

'Oh, *months* back. I sleep here and there. I sleep here when I can't find a floor to sleep on. I'm not doing any harm.'

'You'd better come out. You could get arrested.'

She scrambled out, a curious bundle of disparate garments, hospital white, vaguely Eastern underneath. She said

'It's cold down here. It's hard to keep warm.'

'It's designed to produce an ambient temperature for the Collection, not for squatters.'

Daisy stood up and stared at him.

'I'll go then,' she said, hopefully.

'Where? Where will you go?'

'I'll find somewhere.'

'You'd better come back with me. And sleep in a bed, in a bedroom, if you can bear it.'

'You don't have to sneer.'

'Oh, *for God's sake*, I'm not sneering. Come on.'

Damian cooked pasta, whilst Daisy padded round his flat, studying his prints, with a slightly defiant, assessing look. He found he couldn't ask her what she thought of them. He didn't want to know what she thought of the floods of colour and delicate round harbours of his Herons, the lacquered reds, the gold and orange, the strange floating umber. He put food on the table, and kept the conversation going by asking her questions. He was uneasily aware that his questioning sounded very like a professional medical examination. And that she was answering him because she owed him for the food, the shelter, for not kicking her out of the job or out of the hospital. So he learned that she'd quarrelled with the boyfriend, after and probably because of the complicated abortion. He asked if she'd minded losing the baby, and she said it wasn't a baby, and there was no point in minding or not minding, was there? He asked her if she ate enough, and she said well, what did he *think*, and then recovered her good manners, and said grittily that a hospital was a good place for scrounging, you'd be surprised how much good food went to waste. He asked if she had a grant, or any other source of money than the work at the Collection, and she said no, she did washing-up in restaurants now and then – and office cleaning. She said, economical with the information, that when she got her degree, if she got it, she might think of teaching, but of course that took time up that you might want to spend – need to spend – on your art.

He asked her what sort of work she made, and she said she couldn't say, really, not so he could imagine what it was like. Then she was silent altogether. So he turned on the television – his ex-wife flickered across the scene, playing Beckett, and he changed channels quickly – they watched a football match, Liverpool against Arsenal, and drank a bottle of red wine between them.

In the small hours he heard his bedroom door open, and the pad of footsteps. He slept austerely in a narrow single bed. She came across the room in the dark, like a ghost. She was wearing white cotton panties – he had felt quite unable to offer her any garment to sleep in. She stood and looked down on him, and he looked more or less at the panties, through half-opened eyes. Then she pulled up the corner of the duvet and slid into the bed silently, her cold body pressed against his warm one. Much went through Damian Becket's half-drowsed mind. How he must not hurt her. Not offend her. She put cold fingers on his lips, and then on his sex, which stirred. He touched her, with a gynaecologist's fingers, gently and found the scars of the ovarectomy, a ring pierced into her navel, little breasts with rings in the left nipple. The piercing repelled him. He thought irrelevantly of the pierced hands of the run-of-the-mill man on the cross. She began, not inexpertly, to caress him. He was overcome by a wash of hot emotion – if he had had to name it, he would have called it pity. He took her in his arms, held her to him, made love to her. He felt her tighten and stiffen – thank God there were no more intimate studs or rings – and then she gave a little crow and settled with her head on his chest. He stroked the colourless fluff of her hair in the dark. He said

'You're more a dandelion than a daisy.'

'An old one then, a dead clock.'

That threw him, for he thought of the dispersal of dandelion seeds and then of how inapposite this was to him and her with her ruined tubes. He said

'You know, I have to say, all these studs and things, in soft body tissue – there's a considerable possibility they're carcinogenic.'

'You can't worry about everything,' said Daisy Whimple. 'What a thing to say, at this particular moment.'

'It's what I was thinking.'

'Well, you could keep it to yourself for a better moment.'

'I'm sorry.'

'That's OK.'

He lay on his back, and she lay curled on top of him, and he waited for her to go away, which after a time, perhaps sensing the waiting, she did.

She stayed a week. She came to his bed every night. Every night he stroked the pierced and damaged body, every night he made love to her. At the end of the week she said she'd found a place to go, a friend had a spare sofa. She kissed him for the first time in the daylight, with her clothes on. He felt the cold metal of the ring in her lip. She said, 'I expect you'll be glad to see the back of me. You like your own company, I can see that. But it's been good for you, what we did, for a little bit?'

'Very good.'

'I never know if you mean what you say.'

One result of Daisy's brief habitation was that Damian allowed himself to know that he desired Martha. He wondered briefly if Daisy might have confided in Martha, and concluded that on balance, she would not. He went down to the Collection himself alone, and removed the blankets, the pillows, the food trays. He thought, in a week or so, when his flat was his own again, his sheets were laundered, his solitude with his images re-established, he would invite Martha there. She was a complicated person who needed slow, slow movements, he thought, not really sure why he thought these things. He too needed to move slowly, in a deliberate, considered way, he thought, putting behind him the vision of the white panties, the memory of the metal taste of the nipple-rings.

Martha's behaviour suggested she knew nothing either of Daisy's camp in the Collection, or of the events in Damian's flat. Damian did not mention Daisy to Martha in any context. Martha said she thought she had found an artist-in-residence, a young woman called Sue Basuto.

'I think you'll like her work because it's elegant and colourful and kind of abstract. And I think she'd benefit from a hospital residence because she works with dripping water and pulses of light, in transparent boxes and tubes. She's part of a group show at the St Catherine's Gallery in Wapping. Would you have time to come and look at it? We could perhaps go on and have supper or a drink if you'd like that.'

Damian said he'd like that very much.

They had reached a point where they embraced decorously, cheek to cheek, on meeting and parting.

St Catherine's Gallery turned out to be a cavernous decommissioned red-brick Victorian church, perhaps ten years older than St Pantaleon's Victorian buildings. Damian and Martha went to the opening together: most of the assembled company were art students, some with pink or shocking blue hair. Their voices were small and shrill under the vaulting. They were given transparent plastic beakers of red Australian wine from a winebox, and round potato crisps on plates.

Sue Basuto's work was just inside the door. It had a humming motor, and resembled an Escher woodcut of impossible flow patterns, tipping green floods into crimson funnels over shining slides which balanced finely and reversed the flows. Damian liked it but wondered if it was more than a toy. The people in the church were all gathered to stare at an installation on what had been the altar-steps, under the rood screen. It was hard to see, because of the crowding, and from a distance seemed like a termite heap, or carefully crafted rubbish tip.

Damian and Martha stayed where they were for some time, sipping the wine, which wasn't bad, asking each other whether Sue Basuto's work did or didn't have any reference to the circulation of blood and lymph in the human body. They decided to go and have supper and talk about it. They drifted over to the centre of excitement, before leaving.

*

It was a representation of the goddess Kali, who was constructed like an Arcimboldo portrait out of many elements. She was enthroned in what resembled – what was – a seventeenth-century birthing chair, below which, under the hole into which the baby would drop, was a transparent plastic box full of a jumble of plaster Infants and plaster Mothers from crèches old and new. Kali's black body was a painted écorché sculpture. Her head was a waxwork Vanitas, half smiling lady, half grinning skull, lifesize, crowned with matted ropes of seemingly human hair. Her four arms were medical prostheses, wooden or gleaming mechanical artefacts, ending in sharp steel and blunt wooden fingers, and one hook, from which hung what looked like a real shrunken head, held by the hair. Her earrings were preserved foetuses, decked with beads, enclosed in mahogany-framed glass jars like hourglasses. She brandished a surgical saw in another hand, and the final two arms were crocheting something in an immense tangle of crimson plastic cords. Her crochet hooks were the tools of the nineteenth-century obstetricians, midwives and abortionists; the dreadful formless knitting glittered like fresh blood. She wore, as she traditionally does, a necklace of tiny skulls – apes, rats, humans – and a girdle of dead men's hands, in this case wax clasping plaster of Paris, clasping skeletal fingers clasping what looked like the real thing. Her legs were constructed of interlaced forceps and probes. Her feet were prosthetic – one booted, one a miracle of mechanical joints. She was signed, at her feet, with a flower-shape, a daisy, composed of a circle of the exquisite tiny ivory women round what, on inspection, could be seen to be a yellow contraceptive sponge, about as old as the church.

Damian went white with pure rage.

Martha said 'Oh, how terrible. And how *good*.'

Damian said 'Someone call the police.'

Martha said, 'No, wait – '

The gallery manager, one of the black-clad thin women, came and said, 'What's the problem?'

Daisy sidled up from behind the Kali, just as Damian began to say, very loudly, almost shouting, just controlled, that these objects were valuable museum artefacts – well, and body parts – they were relics and should be treated with respect, they were private property, and their display constituted *theft*. He demanded, he said, that the object be dismantled *immediately*, and the police brought in.

Martha said to the gallery woman, 'He's right. But for God's sake get photos of it before it goes. It's good.'

'It's disgusting,' said Damian. Daisy was standing indecisively, looking as though she was considering the possibility of creeping away through the vestry. He strode up to her and seized her bony little wrist.

'How dare you? How could you? We *trusted you* –'

'I wasn't stealing. I was borrowing.'

'Rubbish. I suppose you would have sold it if you'd had an offer? I hope I never see you again.'

Martha said 'Can't we – discuss...?'

Damian roared '*Get the police!*'

The people slunk away. Daisy twisted free of Damian and began to tear down her structure. Damian shouted that she shouldn't touch the things without gloves, had she learned nothing, she was a little idiot, she seemed to be completely *stupid*, as well as deceitful and hypocritical and *disgusting*...

Martha put her arms round Daisy, who stood shuddering in her grasp for a few minutes, and then twisted free and ran out of the church.

Damian's dinner with Martha did not go as he had planned. He was annoyed by Martha's readiness to praise Daisy's art-work. Martha said it showed real pain, a real sense of human harm, and threats to the female body. Damian said that the reason for this was simply the Things from the Collection, of which she had made an opportunistic use – a *parasitic* use. Damian shouted at Martha as though Martha was Daisy, about the desecration of other people's dead babies and body parts and suffering. Martha said she thought Damian had said that Daisy had lost a baby. That affected people. Damian said she had wanted to lose it, hadn't she, and for his part he didn't think that was why... And why does she haunt the hospital? Martha went on, inexorably. Because she scrounges, I told you, said Damian. Why was Martha so keen on defending a compulsive thief? I'm a woman, said Martha, vaguely and sadly. She had wanted him to notice that, this evening, she had dressed carefully, she had had her hair cut.

The press – luckily only the local press – got hold of the story. SHOCKING 'ARTWORK' 'BORROWED' FROM GRUESOME HOSPITAL RELICS. The Hospital's overworked secretariat fended off queries with talk of a misunderstanding, said all was well that ended well, and said that when eventually the Collection was open to the public, the public would see the true fascination and information value of the relics.

It was probably because of the press stories that Dr Nanjuwany, one of Damian's colleagues, thought of coming to see him. She was a young woman herself, good with patients, still a little nervous with medical difficulties.

'That young woman you were looking after – '

'I wasn't.'

'The one who stole the Things from the Collection. She came to see me.'

Damian closed his face into a simple polite listening.

'She wants an abortion. I looked at her records. She asked for one before, and we made a mess of her, because it turned out to be ectopic. She lost an ovary and most of the tubes. She says she was told she couldn't have any more children and I suspect she was indeed told something of the kind. She worries me. She won't see a counsellor. I feel bad – since the pregnancy is a bit of a miracle – '

'I'll speak to her. Do you have an address?'

'Not really. We tried the one we had – which was the one she gave again when she filled in the forms – and they say she left months ago, they don't know where she is – '

'I want to know when her next appointment is.'

If Dr Nanjuwany was surprised, she hid it. 'Thank you,' she said, as though she meant it.

Damian crept up on Daisy as she sat in the usual long queue in the antenatal clinic.

'I want a word with you,' he hissed, his face rigid with anger. She was sitting with the dandelion head bowed down, staring into her lap. She looked up at him whitely.

'No, thank you.'

'It's not "yes please" or "no thank you", Daisy, it's stand up *now* and come with me. *Now.*'

'You can't hit me.'

'Don't be silly. I'm trying to help.'

'That's not what you look like you're doing.'

'That's because I'm also upset. I'm human. Now, come and talk this over, in private, come into my office.'

She sat there in his office, facing him, where all his patients sat. She said

'I've done nothing wrong.'

'Well, apart from theft, and unlawful entry, no. I want to talk to you about the baby.'

'It's not a baby, right. It's a problem. It's got no future. We all know that, so just fuck off, OK?'

'Whose baby is it?'

'It's *not a baby.* The last one wasn't, it was a life-threatening *incubus,* that's what it was. Nearly killed me.'

'Whose baby is it?'

'Whose do you think it is? That's all you men care about, nice potent sperm, sod the consequences – '

'Shut up, Daisy. If this is my baby – and it is a baby, it's a minor miracle – then I can't just let you destroy it – like that, without thinking.'

'You don't know if I think or not. You don't know nothing about me. You can't call this a *relationship,* nobody ever pretended it was. It was a bit of fun and it went wrong. So I'm dealing with it in a grown-up way, a *responsible* way, to use Dr-Becket-think. It's not your body, it's nothing to do with you now. So get out of my life.'

'It's my baby. It is my body. It's turning into my flesh and blood in there. You're not going to kill it.'

'Very nice. And who will look after it, once it's got here, if it hasn't killed me and itself on the way?'

'I will, that's obvious. I'll support you – whilst you wait – and take the baby – and find a way to look after him. Or her.'

'You would, wouldn't you? Shit. Get it adopted into a *nice* family, keep an eye on its progress...'

'It's my child. It should be with me. Fathers do love their children.'

'Not unborn ones, in my experience. And I don't have no father, so I wouldn't know.'

'They don't love unborn ones mostly because they don't imagine them. I deliver them all the time – especially those in trouble – so I do imagine them.'

A generic howling newborn crossed his overactive mental imagery. He said 'I'm sorry you have no father. Is he dead?'

'I just don't know who he is. I grew up in a commune. My mother was in a kind of East London ashram thing. All the men were meant to be fathers to all the kids. They weren't, not really. They all, like, went their own way and did their own thing after a year or two.'

'So you lived with your mother?'

'No, she died. I lived a bit with my gran, but she went a bit crazy and got put into a place where they put crazy people, and I went to one of the other commune women, but she went to India, so I got fostered, like, with a teacher, which was the family I had, but I'm not in touch any more... Is this an interrogation?'

'No. I wanted to know. I don't mean to shout. I want my child to be born. If you can bear it.'

'That's a joke.'

'It wasn't meant to be. I can and will look after you. – '

'No, but I like my own life, doing my own things my own way ...'

'Daisy, please. It might be your only chance... to have...'

'Do you think I *don't know that*?'

*

Hospital consultants are used to getting their way. Daisy wriggled and argued. Damian simply heard her out and restated his position. She left, saying she would 'think about it when you're not screaming at me'. He said he would write her a cheque to buy food and Daisy enquired what good he thought *that* would do, since she had no bank account. So he emptied out the cash from his pockets, and put it into hers, as she sat there, sullen and silent. She said 'This looks pretty disgusting. *I* think.'

'You've got to eat. For two.'

'That remains to be seen.'

'Where are you living?'

'Here and there. Nowhere you could find me.'

'Please. Promise to keep in touch. You will need looking after. Properly.'

She said in a tired whisper

'OK. I promise.'

He said nothing of this to Martha Sharpin. He was a doctor, he had taken the Hippocratic Oath, silence came easy to him. But what he was not saying inhibited him from saying anything else. He didn't call her. Then Martha, like Dr Nanjuwany, knocked at his office door. They kissed, cool cheek to cool cheek.

'Damian, I've had a surprising visit. From Daisy.'

'Oh?'

'She turned up very late last night and asked if she could sleep on my floor. So I said yes, and she came in, and just started crying – I've never seen anyone cry so much – and it all came out. Or a lot of it. She said you are insisting she doesn't have an abortion, and she wants an abortion, but she can't answer you back because you're so overbearing. And I wondered if a baby was in her interest – was possible for her – really. She's turned me into a kind of proxy mother. So I thought I'd come and ask you directly – since she's still on my sofa, and shows no sign of leaving – '

'The baby is in *my* interest,' said Damian.

'But you are a *lapsed* Catholic, you said so.'

'Seeing it's *my baby* – '

He saw, from Martha's face, that Daisy had for some reason been more discreet, or secretive, than he could possibly have hoped.

'Oh,' said Martha. Damian said

'I was trying to be kind. I was only trying to be kind.'

He could not read Martha's expression. Shock, censure, disappointment, puzzlement.

'I found her camping out in the basement. I took her home. She got in my bed. It would have been damnably *rude* somehow to kick her out, somehow. You know. No, you don't.'

'Oh, we've all gone to bed with people because it would have been rude not to.' A little too lightly. 'So now what?'

'Well. I – I shall take the baby. She needn't see it, she clearly doesn't want it, but it must be *born*. I'm responsible for it. What a mess.'

They stared at each other. Damian, domineering with Daisy, was hangdog with Martha. Martha said 'She really is miserable. She's twisting about like an octopus on a fish-hook. What about her – medical problems? Will it be straightforward? She's scared stiff.'

'Possibly it won't. Won't be straightforward. I don't know. There are very clear rights and wrongs in this matter.'

'Possibly there are, in your head,' said Martha.

'You don't agree? You don't see – how I see it – what I feel?'

'Not exactly. I'm an outsider. I see what she wants, and I see what you want. The two don't fit very well.'

There appeared to be no room at all for what Martha herself might want, or have wanted.

'I need to find her somewhere to live – in a sensible way – or as near sensible as possible. Not your sofa.'

'Not my sofa. I'm not a saint and I have my own life. I'll put my mind to the problem of lodging.'

'I'll pay.'

'Oh yes,' said Martha. 'I understand that.'

*

A room was found, in a reasonable bed and breakfast, not far from where Martha lived, in London Fields. Martha helped in the search for the room and put a glass of freesias on the little dressing table. She also helped Daisy to move in, in Damian's absence. She reported back to Damian that Daisy had said almost nothing, and didn't look well. She seems beaten down, said Martha to Damian. Defeated. She thought for a moment and added inexorably, 'Terrified.' Damian said frigidly that Martha was not to worry. It was his problem, and his decision, and he would see to it, and he was grateful for her help, and promised not to bother her any further. They looked at each other unhappily. Daisy now bulked large in both their minds; she had made them into the parents she didn't have, setting the kind mother against the domineering father, and herself against both. Life runs in very narrow stereotyped channels, until it is interrupted by accidents or visions. Daisy somehow impeded Damian and Martha from becoming lovers as a small child nightly interrupts its parents' embraces. Damian had this thought rather grimly as he drove to the hospital. He had the further thought that Daisy's real child – his child – when it was born, would be an even more effective impediment.

He oversaw Daisy's pregnancy in a manner both cunning and draconian. He knew better than to invade her private life – or work life, whatever that was. But he checked what he knew about. He made sure she kept all her appointments, he monitored her monitoring, he checked the prescriptions, he interrogated Dr Nanjuwany. He set his mind to thinking what to do with a baby. He did not consult Martha, he did not consult Dr Nanjuwany. He did have a conversation with the hospital almoner, about what the legal processes were in the case of babies that were to be given up for adoption. This area turned out to be murky and fraught with difficulty. He listened to the almoner about the rights of the mother, the lack of rights of the father, about adoption procedures for a putative father who wanted an unwanted child. The simplest would be to marry, said the almoner. Not possible, said Damian. Damian, naturally law-abiding, and troubled about the legal status of his unborn child, nevertheless decided by default simply to do what was best and sort out a de facto situation later. He found out about nanny agencies.

He was subjected, over the remaining months of gestation, to a kind of martyrdom by whispering. Everyone 'knew' what was going on, and since neither Damian, nor, surprisingly, Daisy, confided in anyone, guesswork and innuendo flourished and tangled. Daisy did go so far as to report stonily that she didn't want the baby, and didn't want to be told how it was getting on, she wasn't keeping it, it was all someone else's business, thank you. Damian was present when the first ultrasound pictures of the child, stirring in its fluid bath, appeared on the screen. Daisy turned her face away. Dr Nanjuwany said 'Do you want to know the sex or not? Some people like to be surprised.'

Damian said, 'It's a girl. I can see her. She's fine.'

Daisy said 'You, Dr Becket, will you *go away*, please.'

He interviewed nannies. They came and sat on his sofa in his elegant flat, and stared at his paintings. He told them that the newborn baby would arrive in three months, and that it was his own baby whose mother would be unable to care for her. They stared with a child-carer's pity at the pale upholstery. One, who was friendly, and the eldest of seven – 'I've looked after kids since I was twelve years old, I know all their ways...' he rejected because she was Irish, and wore a religious medal. One, very upper class, had a slightly loopy look and said she didn't think Docklands was a very suitable place to bring up a baby. They need fresh air, she said, looking as though finding even these words was a disagreeable effort to her. He didn't like the sensation of being about to be dependent on, in need of placating, these unknown young women. He finally picked a Dane, called Astrid, largely because she knew about painting, exclaimed over the Herons and the Terry Frosts, said, without pushing, that it would be good for a child to grow up amidst such colour.

*

Daisy nearly lost the baby at seven months. She was in the hospital for a week, with symptoms of pre-eclampsia, curious pillows of swollen flesh growing around her stick-like ankles. Damian visited her every day. He checked up on her body, and his child's body inside her body. She didn't really talk to him any more. The defiance had gone out of her, and was replaced by an unnerving combination of resignation and fear. When Damian said the foetus was in a good position, or that her blood pressure had improved, she said, 'Well, that's good, then,' as though she expected nothing, neither good nor bad.

If Martha visited Daisy, Damian didn't see her. He had seen Martha drive away from the hospital with a man – a man in a good mohair suit, with longish hair, talking animatedly. Martha had her own life. He had a wife in Ireland and an unborn baby in Pondicherry Ward.

But it was to Martha that Daisy ran when her waters broke, unexpectedly early. Martha, mistrustful of ambulances, put Daisy in her own car and drove her to St Pantaleon's. Daisy, her body heaving, her face blue-white, said 'Don't go away, please don't go away.'

The admissions desk alerted Dr Nanjuwany, who took it on herself to alert Damian. He came down to find Daisy clutching Martha's clothes, saying, 'Don't go away. Please don't go away.' Martha looked at Damian. She thought there must be some ethical reason why he should not be involved in what was about to happen. She observed that he was at the end of some tether, his self-control exaggerated absurdly. She said, 'No, I won't go away. I want to see this baby.'

Daisy said, 'There won't be no baby. It will all go wrong. I've known that all along.' She howled, very loudly, over a wave of contraction and pain 'It's going to die and so am I and *he* knows it is, and he knows I am, *he* knows...'

Martha said to Damian, as Daisy was wheeled away

'She's in pain. She doesn't mean what she says – '

'Yes, she does.'

'They say women in labour shout out all sorts of things...'

'They do. I know, it's my job. But she does think she's going to die. I see it now. I didn't see it before. She's the sort of person I can't – I can't imagine what she really thinks or feels – *at all*.'

'Would it be all right if I stay?'

'It isn't your problem.'

'She came to me.'

And *I didn't*, he wanted to cry. Exactly because... He wanted to cry, *I* didn't. Exactly because she did I couldn't. And can't. He flipped his mind back to obstetrics.

'I need to check how she's doing,' he said.

Daisy's labour was long and horrible. She made it worse by letting loose nine months of pent-in terror and rage, screaming, weeping, and tensing all her muscles. She could not be anaesthetised too much, for fear of harming the baby, whose heartbeat was irregular, whose presentation turned out to be very awkward, with a twisted shoulder. Dr Nanjuwany in turn panicked and, ignoring what she knew and had not been told were all the ethical reasons for not involving Damian, turned to him. He ended up delivering a live baby, slowly, deliberately, skilfully, not because he was its father, but because he was the man at that moment in that hospital who could deal with such a problem. He stitched the dangerous rip in the neck of Daisy's womb, stroked the pale hair away from the sodden forehead, took her pulse, and wondered where her wandering soul was drifting as she relaxed into a drugged and unencumbered peace. He had nearly killed her. That was the truth of it.

He went to look at his daughter.

She had been washed, and swaddled, and was breathing lightly, regularly. She had soft dark hair. She was a little bruised. She opened hazy mussel-dark eyes, and seemed to consider him. He looked back at her, not in pride at his achievement – although in the melodramatic way of real lives, he had saved her, and indeed Daisy. He was overcome with dreadful love and grief. She was a person. She had not been there, and now she was there, and she was the person he loved. It was simple and he was a changed man. His eyes were hot with tears. The hospital rustled and whispered behind him.

When he went to visit the next day, he found he was in the grip of an exalted fear. He was going to see the child again – that was the essential thing. In his mind he had named her Kate. He was going to see Daisy, who did not want to know or see Kate. He thought he would start with the difficult thing – he was not a procrastinator – the difficult thing was Daisy. Then he would revisit his daughter.

Daisy was in a curtained-off space of her own, with a bowl of fruit on her locker. She was sitting up in bed in a hospital nightshirt, and her hair was washed and floating. She was holding – he saw her – the baby, in her arms, at her breast. The baby was feeding. He could see the little ripples of movement in the fine skin over the back of her skull. She was feeding from the pierced nipple. Daisy's little face was completely wet with tears. Her little hands, with their tattooed mittens, tightened round Kate, and grasped. She stared at Damian as though he meant to rip the child out of her arms. Her lip, with its silly studs, trembled.

Damian sat down heavily on the visitor's chair. Daisy said, in a small but perfectly grown-up voice

'I didn't understand. I didn't know. She's perfect. No, it isn't that, everybody says that. She's *somebody*, she's a person, and she's mine and she – seems to need me. I mean, it does seem to be *me* she needs. I mean, I can't help it, she can't help it, I'm – hers, I mean, I'm her mother.' The word obviously gave her trouble. She repeated. 'I didn't understand. I didn't know.'

Damian said 'You are right of course. She is also mine.' He could have added 'And I am hers,' but he wasn't capable of so much rhetoric.

'You know, they all go on about love. Love, love, love. You and me, me and you – well, not you and me *personally*, but in the abstract. No one writes songs to babies, do they? But when I *saw* her – that was love, that was *it*, I know what it is – '

'I know. That's what I felt. When I saw her.'

The baby hiccupped. Awkwardly, but gently, Daisy tipped her up on her shoulder and patted her back. Then, gingerly, she held her out to Damian, who took her in his arms, and looked down into the unique, lovely face.

'What the hell are we going to do now?' Damian asked.

Martha, bringing a posy of daisies and anemones, came into the little space to find them both staring at the child, who lay on her shawl on the bed between them. Damian and Daisy had faces of baffled adoration. Daisy was still weeping, steadily and easily. It was perfectly clear to Martha what had happened. She thought of walking away, quickly. Damian repeated, just as he caught sight of Martha

'What the hell are we going to do now?'

Daisy said to Martha, like a child to its mother,

'I didn't understand. I didn't know.'

'Don't cry,' said Martha, coming further in. She saw that Damian had tears in his eyes. The baby began to cry and Damian and Daisy both put out their arms to pick her up and comfort her, and both drew back together. Martha, not herself moved to adoration, could see no satisfactory way out of this state of affairs, which was supposed to be not her problem.

'We'll think of something. Because we shall have to,' she said. The other two nodded vaguely. All three continued to stare at the baby.

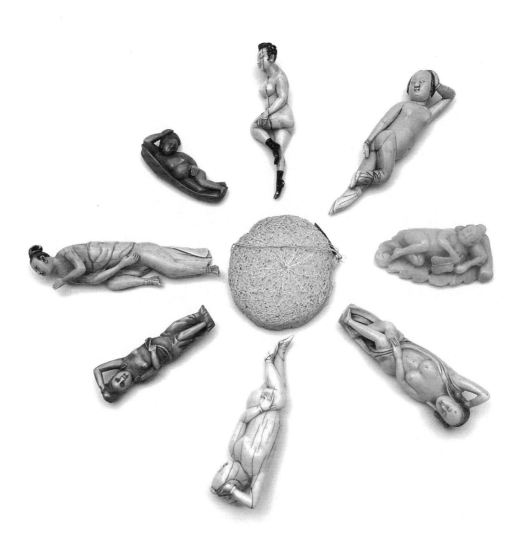

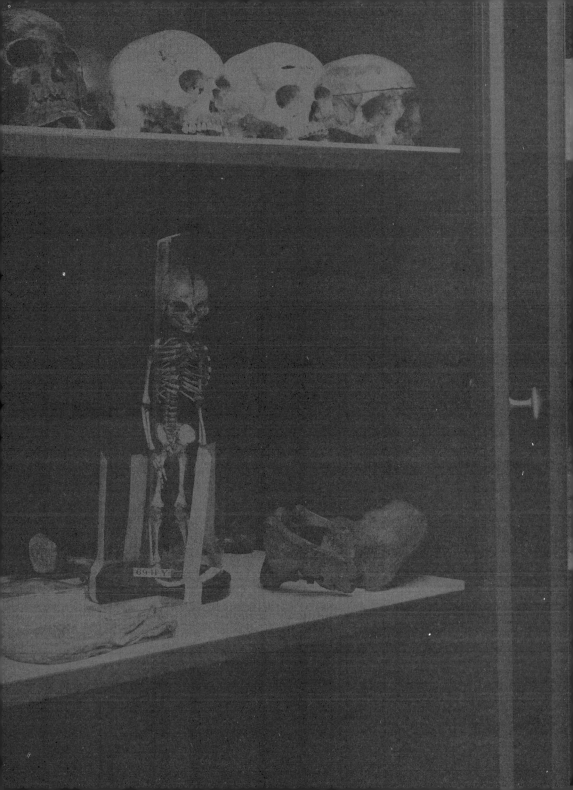

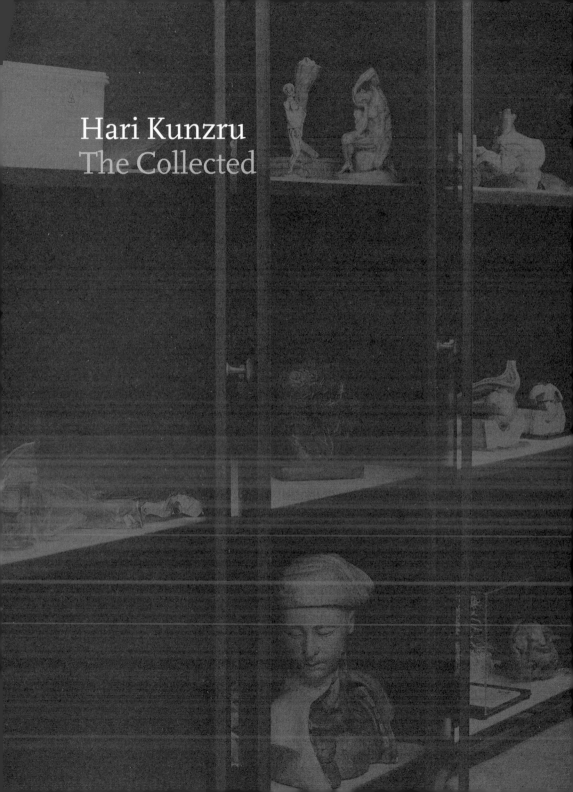

Hari Kunzru
The Collected

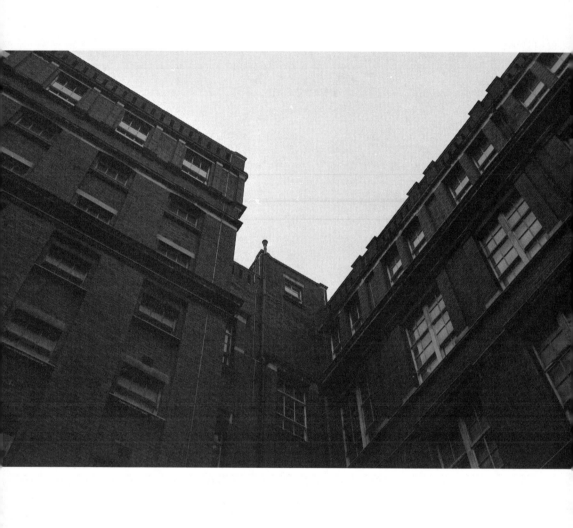

It is dark in here.

In the corridors where your feet strike sharp little notes on the tiles.

In the rooms filled with rows of numbered metal racks. Cabinets and drawers.

There are procedures to ensure the staff do not get locked in, trapped behind the electronic security, the heavy doors. At least one of them believes in ghosts. He would not like to spend the night here, alone in the dark.

But I am here.

There are others too.

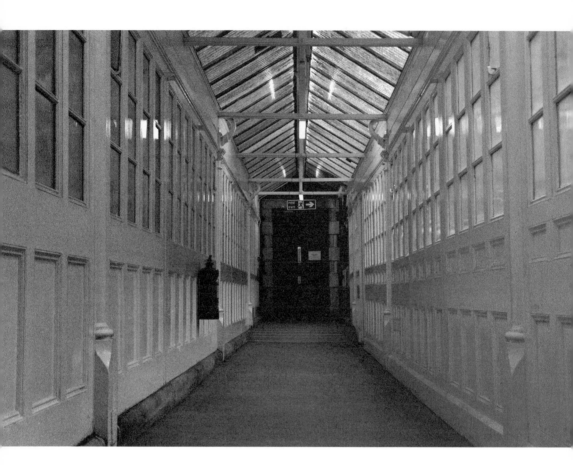

Institutionalised, that's me.

The collector had to have old Thomson's machine. And some examples of what it could do. I came with it so to speak. A single tear on a notebook page. That's all it takes.

I cried. I admit it. More than once. Out of frustration mostly.

> *Is it too much to hope that at least in British territory the night is finally gone. & that under enlightened & sympathetic rule the Negro will now have an opportunity of developing him_self & his country?   For a period of transition has arrived in earnest? the misionary the goverment and tyhe railway in   very diverse ways are creating a new west africa making it difficult to   write in the   present tense of fashions that flourished ten years ago.*

When I finished it the doctor said well done and took the page away and wrote underneath *typed by William Witt (who has no arms) by means of the perfected model of the 'Mechanical Substitute for the arms' which is used for instruction at Roehampton Hospital.*

It was a marvel, they said.

A miracle.

Roll up, roll up.

Watch the armless man smoke a cigarette!
Watch him eat meat with a knife and fork!
Watch him drink tea!

All with his feet. Thanks to Thomson's table, with its levers and snap grips and racks of metal tools.

They were all brim-full of ambition. Mrs Gwynne-Holford and her hospital. Thomson and his bloody contraption. All except me. They tried to gee me up, told me I had to make an effort. But I couldn't see the point. Not of writing. Not of anything in a world like this. A world in which things like the war could happen.

There were forty-one thousand of us by the end. And even with all them armless and legless boys on the streets people still couldn't look me in the eye. Two little flaps just below my shoulders is what I had to work with. Like a penguin. Couldn't have held my kids if I had any. Couldn't have held my girl if I still had her. But I sat there and they fitted me into Thomson's table and I knuckled down and did a bit out of the paper. A whole paragraph. The doctor leaned over and wrote his comment and said look on the bright side, now the generals can make you into a clerk and send you back. Then he took the page of typing and put it in my file.

Took me the best part of an hour.

Is it too much to hope that at least in British territory the
night is finally gone, & that under enlightened & sympathetic
rule the Negro will now have an opportunity of developing him_
self & his country? For a period of transition has arrived
in earnest? the misionary the goverment and tyhe railway in
very diverse ways are creating a new west africa making it
difficult to write in the present tence of fashions that
flourished ten yers ago.

*Typed by William Witt (who has no arms)
by means of the perfected model of the
"Mechanical Substitute for the arms"
which is used for instruction at Rockampton
Hospital.*

AC023.21

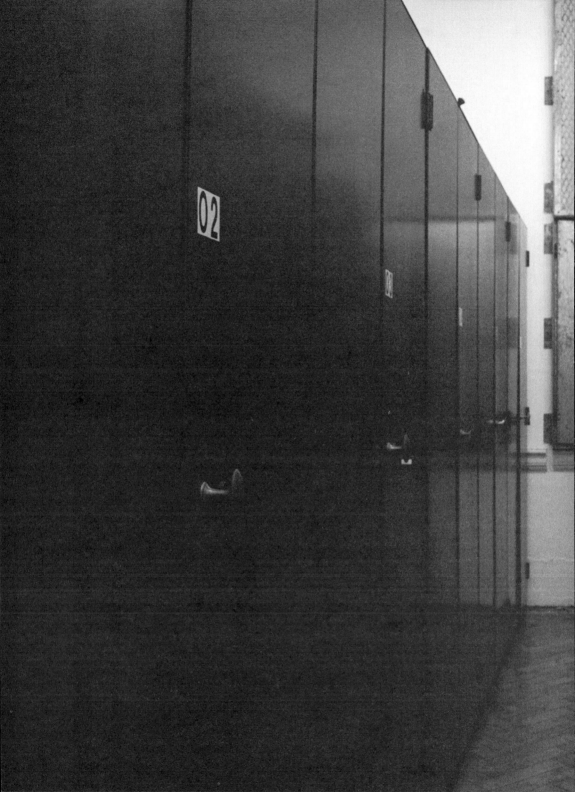

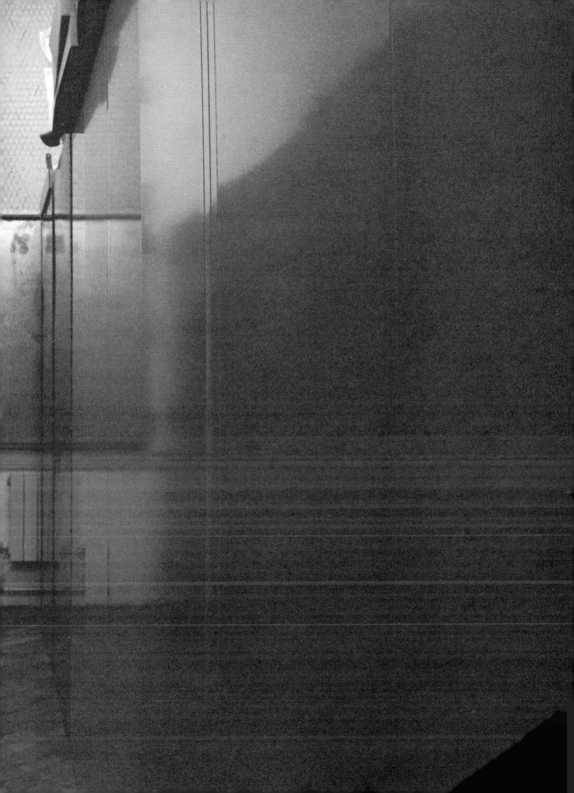

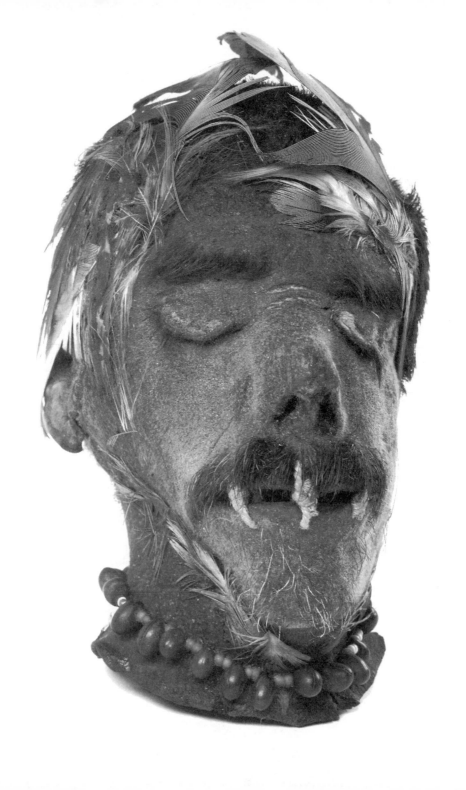

Me?

Why am I here?

Gold, of course. What else would be the reason?

I was once Juan Ignacio Perez-Santos, out of Havana. Now I
am just Juan the Idiot, head blackened and shrunk to the size
of an orange, lips neatly sewn up with thick fibrous string.
Why? Because I dreamed of gold and women and an end to
working on the ships.

The collector bought my head from a Frenchman, who in turn
had it from a mestizo trader, who swapped it with the Jivaro for
two elderly bolt action rifles. Two, you understand. Not one.
The head of Juan the Idiot is a rarity.

My life had a gradual southerly drift. From Havana down
through the Caribbean, port by port. In Belize I fell ill. In
Martinique I won money and almost stayed. In Panama City I
had a wife, who left me. After that I signed on as second mate
of a steamer bound for Ecuador. In Esmeraldas, in a cantina
where the patron stood on a ladder nailing a picture of the new
president of the Republic above the bar I met a man who told
me a story about gold. We drank aguardiente and he made a
flickering motion with his fingers, like coins falling towards
the tabletop. How will you ever become rich unless you take a
chance, he asked. He said other things such as *the only men
who deserve their dreams are the ones who have the courage to
grasp them.* Fine words. *Grasp them.* The hands clenching tight,
pulling meaning out of the air. I drank aguardiente and the
sweat stood out in beads on my face and I agreed to go upriver
to seek gold and be one of those men who deserves his dreams.

First you have to sever the head. Then you cut a slit at the back, and with knives and spatulas ease the scalp and the fleshy part of the face away from the skull. After that you can do what you like with the skull; the Jivaro threw mine into the river to placate the anaconda spirit. Now carefully turn the face inside out and scrape off the fatty tissue. When you have cleaned the thin sheet of skin, which should be almost translucent, you must simmer it in water and herbs. Not boil, mind. Just simmer. The thing will disintegrate if the liquid gets too hot. Then sew up the back of the neck, the eyes and the lips. The rest is done with heat, hot pebbles and sand inside the little head-sack, the skin shrinking and hardening, the features emerging as you reshape them with your hands. Finally, when the head is as small and light and hard as you can make it, you dye it black with a paste made from charcoal, and start on the rituals which will allow you to transfer the head's spiritual power to yourself.

So we canoed up the river with two metal trunks of trade goods. Knife blades and cooking pots, new carbines wrapped in oiled cloth, boxes of ammunition. The hot green pulse of the forest thickened the air, which became heady and stifling, hard to take down into your lungs. We travelled for weeks, pushing ourselves up the silent brown river, drinking gulps of brackish water which seemed to seep back out of the skin before the cap was even on the canteen.

We had a piece of paper. On it was a map, and directions to the country of the Shuar, who did not know the value of gold – or so at least claimed the man who sold the map to my friend. Idiot Juan never thought to ask about this man, his name, whether he appeared richly dressed. Had he been to the Shuar to take gold for himself? It does not matter now, but I suspect I

know the answer. Neither of us could read, yet we believed
in the paper. When we took it out to look at, we thought that
we could see ourselves, our little canoe, somewhere along
the scratched line of blue ink.

It is a stupid story, really. There is nothing to it. We canoed
upriver. We talked of gold. For food we shot sloths and
roasted them over the fire. One evening as we tied up to the
bank, the Shuar, who do not care much for gold but are fond
of territory and manioc beer and heads, came for ours.
There was a sound, a sharp exhalation from the forest, and
then a tiny clattering on the gunwales of the boat. I felt a
stinging pain on my face and neck, and putting up my hand
I touched a dart, which stood out of my throat like a little
flagpole. As we struggled in the half-light for our guns, I
tripped and fell into the water. It was not deep but the
bottom was a sucking tangle of mud and creepers. I tried to
stand but kept stumbling. As I flailed about on my hands
and knees, trying to hold my breath, I felt someone in the
water behind me. Then my head was jerked up by the hair
and I cleared the surface and took a gulp of air which all at
once became a gurgle of blood.

There, in a few words, is the story of Juan the Idiot, who
believed the stories he was told in bars. Juan who paddled
upriver and got his throat cut. There are Jivaro here, Shuar
and others, who believe humans have their origins with the
sloths. We are closer kin than we like to admit. I wonder,
was I just a fool? Or is this punishment for something
more than stupidity?

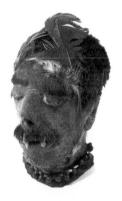

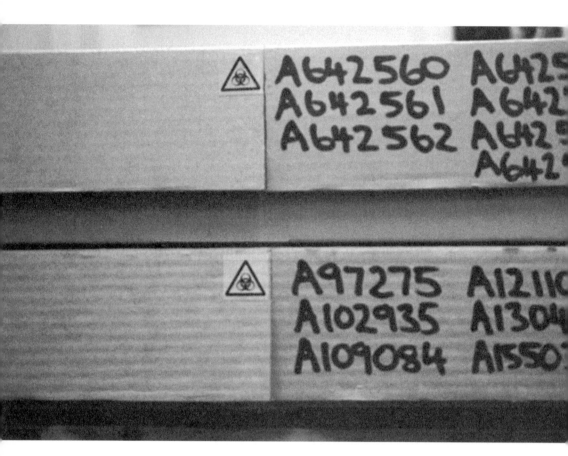

He was not an artistic man, my lover. He had to pay someone
else to do the work, to take the lock of my hair and tease it
into these little representations of ferns and willows. I do not
hold that against him. Some men are good with their hands.
Some, like my lover, must rely on other things. So when he
had finished weeping he lifted his face from my cold fingers,
took the gold-handled scissors from my sewing box and cut
my hair. Then he wrapped the hair in tissue paper and tied it
with a piece of ribbon from the sewing box and took it to the
Jew who kept the jeweller's shop in the market square.

The jeweller, who was a compassionate man, had to coax my
lover into giving up his relic. He guessed what was going
through his mind, why he stood at the counter trembling,
unable to hand it over. The doubt about bringing me to a Jew,
about a Jew's dirty hands on my golden hair. The jeweller
understood, saw that here was yet another humiliation to
store among the clutter in his life. He knew that he inspired
disgust and – this is amazing to me – still cleared a space in
which to feel pity for his customer. The jeweller swallowed
his anger and found sadness and with it a voice in which to
say words of sympathy, to promise to do the work well for the
young gentleman. And my lover let go of his disgust and
passed the little packet across the counter.

Love is a sickness. Love can also be a kind of theatre played
out for the beloved. Day after day during my illness my lover
performed at my bedside. As I tried not to cough he
demonstrated his anguish, showing forth his sufferings like
a sickroom Garrick. He sighed and wiped away his tears,
never letting me forget that although I was facing my death,
he too was in pain. My troubles would end. His would carry
on. His mourning and loneliness. My blessed release. He

insisted on nursing me, would fuss at the bedclothes and spill things. While I could speak I attempted to comfort him. Later I simply tried not to feel irritated.

He did not know what he wanted done with it. The jeweller suggested a locket, and showed him a piece of work he had made for someone else. My lover thought it good, but wanted his memento to be finer, to confirm that his love and thus his loss were greater than the other man's. The jeweller suggested willow trees, drooping over a little tomb. He named a price. I will say one thing; my lover did not try to bargain. He was a proud man and had a sense of the dignity of a transaction. For two years after the locket was finished he wore it on a ribbon round his neck. Later, after he was married, he kept it in a locked drawer of his writing desk.

Now when I think of love, I think of hands. I think of the jeweller's delicate hands, taking strands of my hair and teasing them into the shape of trees. Hands, patient and tender, arranging everything in place, painting on the side of the tomb a little unbelieved-in Christian cross. Even now that I am here, the property of the collector, I am marked by the touch of those hands. Perhaps, had I been loved by a man more like the jeweller, my life would have been different. Perhaps I would have felt more.

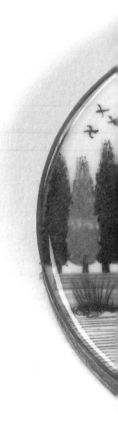

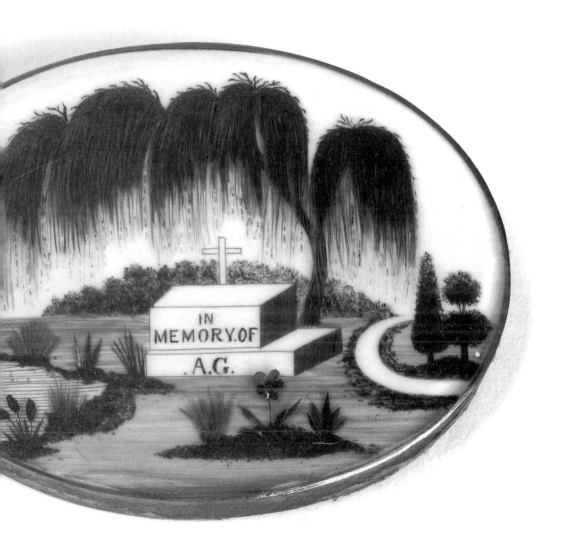

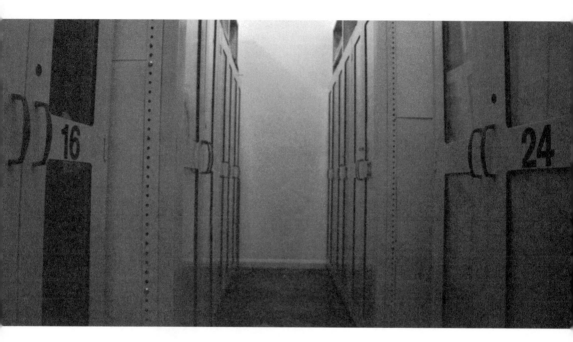

How many skulls, marked in how many ways? The terrifying Maori savage, rudely carved with the diabolical leering forms they call 'tiki'. The Oriental monk they made into a rather tasteless cup. The cranium signed by a whole anatomy class. Imagine it, spending eternity in the form of a college memento! How depressing! How deeply *démodé*!

I like to think that I made a contribution to the natural sciences, though perhaps that merely means I have a distended organ of hope. You can confirm this if you like. My own skull is conveniently marked with the location of the part of the brain which governs this quality, as well as that of the other thirty-six mental and moral faculties. They are, you will recall from your studies:

Amativeness
Philoprogenitiveness
Adhesiveness
Combativeness
Destructiveness
Secretiveness
Acquisitiveness
Self esteem
Approbativeness
Cautiousness
Individuality
Locality
Form
Verbal memory
Language
Colouring
Tune
Calculativeness
Constructiveness
Comparison
Causality
Wit
Ideality

Benevolence
Imitativeness
Generation
Firmness
Time
Eventuality
Inhabitiveness
Reverence
Conscientiousness
Marvellousness
Size
Weight and resistance
and
Order

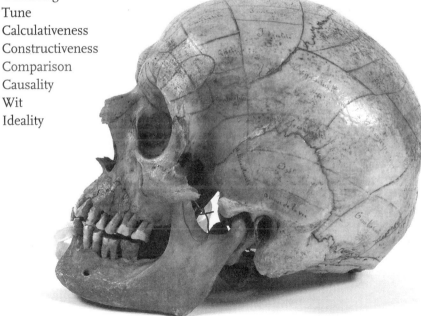

Not that I was ever a man of any great learning. My scientific career was an entirely post-mortem affair. Galvanising frogs' legs? Killing sparrows in vacuum chambers? Goodness me, no. I was possessed of a sensibility more romantic than rational. At the zenith of my admittedly undistinguished progression through life I kept a shop in Piccadilly, the same shop into which I had been apprenticed at thirteen years of age. That was in the days when the quality wore wigs, and I had grown up in a haze of starch powder, threading human hair in a stink of lavender and orange and orris root. By the time I was one and twenty my hands were crossed-hatched with burns from curling tongs and I could fashion false hair into the most extravagant and fantastical confections. Ships at sea. Cloudscapes. I was, I like to flatter myself, something of an artist.

When I was five and twenty my master died, and since he was what might delicately be termed a confirmed bachelor (that is to say one who always preferred the molly-houses of Covent Garden to any kind of settled domesticity) I found myself his sole heir. Such was my pleasure in my good fortune that, I am sorry to say, I went quite wild. I neglected first my books, then my customers and finally made the cardinal error, fatal in a person of my occupation, of losing touch with the fashion. As gentlemen and ladies began to wear their natural hair, I was too preoccupied with cards and porter to fret, assuming that this was a fad, and the following season the pendulum would swing back towards the perruque.

That error of judgement placed my life on a short and perilously steep downhill path.

As the periwig vanished permanently from the heads of the London gentry, my livelihood vanished with it. I fell into debt, then into despair, and finally headfirst into a gallon jar of gin. When I reached the bottom, my shop gone, my mind a blur, my hands too shaky to tie a knot or wield a pair of shears, the Marshalsea was all that awaited me. There, amidst the squalor and the vermin, I spent long years watching my body decline. I was once a well-favoured youth, possessed of a finely turned leg and a profile that was once termed 'romanesque' by no lesser personage than Lord Kenyon, an occasional customer of my master. By the time the anatomist purchased my corpse from the gaoler all this had long gone. Vanity! I was a bag of bones, barely fit for the scalpel. Most of my body eventually found its way into the Cross Bones graveyard in Southwark, but my skull went into the anatomist's collection, where it stayed, locked in a cupboard, for many years. At length, with the rise of the phrenological theories of Doctor Gall, it was marked out with the good German's divisions of the mental faculties and converted, much to my pleasure, into a teaching aid.

Those were my glory days. I was handled, scrutinised, debated and argued over in a most flattering manner. I was most disappointed when the doctor's theories were superseded. People had the nerve to call him a charlatan! Worse, I was pronounced tasteless. Tasteless, me? In a way, I was rather relieved to be purchased by the collector. I am part of something permanent, something that does not change with the seasons. For (alas!) I believe it will always be my fate to fall out of fashion.

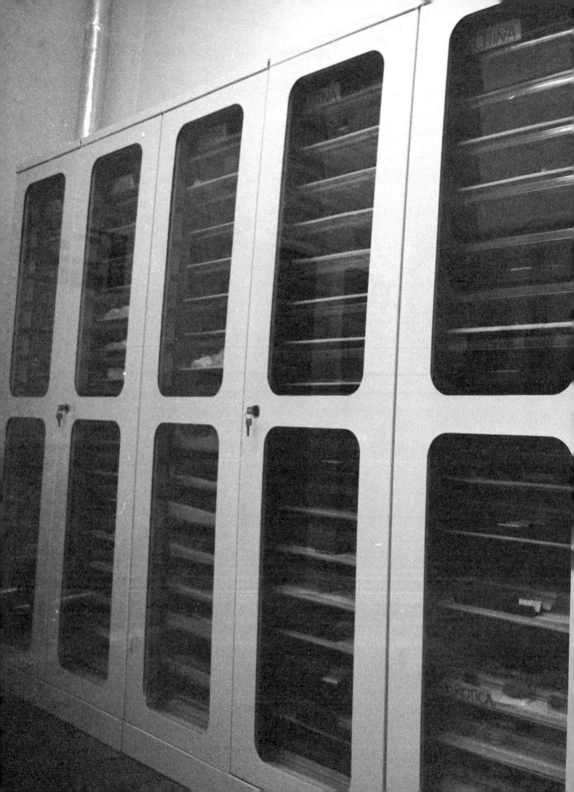

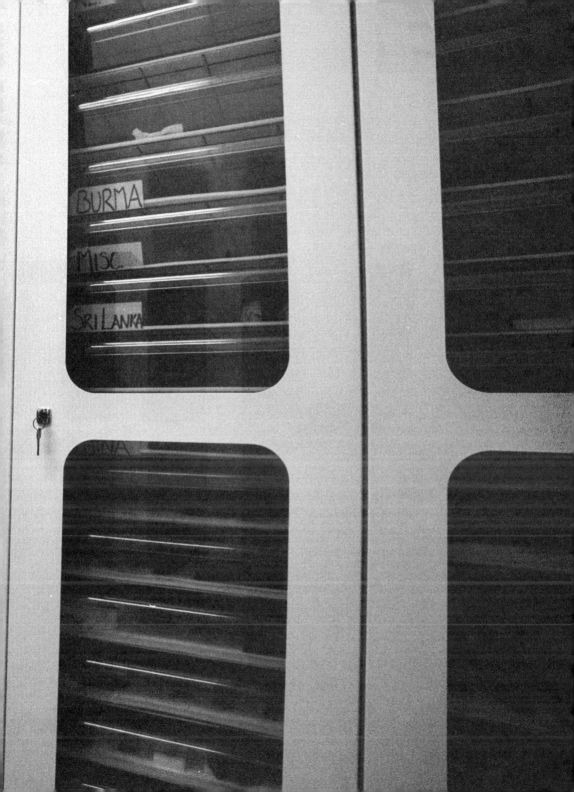

What you can't tell is that I'm a woman. You could in life
though. The boys certainly had no problem. Sometimes I
thought their eyes would fall out of their heads. I liked it. I
always enjoyed attention.

When I was a young girl I earned a living how I could. Later I
kept a place on the waterfront. The Red Dog. It was my pride
and joy, a little scrap of a bar with good food and a floor that
was usually in need of a mop. It was my place, bought with
my own money, and though a lot of the men who came in
there fancied themselves as the lord and master, none of
them ever got close. Not until Jules. After him there could be
no one else. He was my beginning and my end, and he was a
jealous man. More than one of my admirers came away
bleeding for having spoken out of turn, or looking too
intently at me over the zinc counter.

The company at The Red Dog was not what you would call
respectable. At least once a week the police would come
through the door looking for someone. Sometimes they were
looking for Jules. I was always scared I would lose him that
way, that one or other of his crimes would be found out.
People said he was mad, and even in the early days I was
aware he had a temper. But I liked a man who knew his
mind, and I loved to run my hands over his body and trace
the pictures tattooed there. He had pictures from all over the
world, from Japan and Sumatra and Hong Kong and San
Francisco. There was writing too, oaths and promises. He
had kept a record of his whole life on his skin. On one arm he
had 'je jure de me venger' and a skull, which was for the
judge who put him in Mettray colony when he was only a boy.
On his chest just above his heart was something which was
truer than he knew. 'J'ai mal commencé, je finirais mal.'

You expect to feel the back of their hand once in a while, and
that's how it was for the first few years. If he thought I'd
been flirting with the customers, or I questioned where he'd
been. The way I saw it, to have such a storybook of a man
was worth a few bruises. Keys and hearts and teardrops and
crosses. Sailing ships and ladies in kimonos. Life had taught
me that nothing good comes without pain, and Jules was
magnificent. A real man, the rage bottled up inside him so
you felt you might get burned just by standing too close.

But he began to brood. He would ask do you love me how
much do you love me tell me how much. I said I would do
anything, would give anything, and he sat there in the
parlour wearing clothes I had bought for him, scowling and
saying prove you love me. So I told him we were for life. I
told him I would show him. And one morning while he was
still sleeping it off I went to Paul's barbers in the Rue
Paradis and spoke to Paul about what I wanted done. At first
Paul would not hear of it, but I showed him money, and he
took me into the back room.

Afterwards, when it was still bloody and raw, I ran to show
Jules. He rubbed his eyes and stared at his own face, his
portrait inked on my skin over my heart. Then he cried and
slapped and embraced me and screamed and one thing
turned into another over and over until I didn't know what
was pain and what was love and I didn't care.

In the long term the tattoo didn't change things. Maybe it
even made them worse. Something was broken. He had
stopped trusting me. Sometimes he hit me so hard I fell
unconscious. I got so scared. He believed all kinds of things.
I thought he would kill me. Then one night he came at me

while I was chopping vegetables for dinner. One of the girls
found me the next morning, sitting on the floor with the
knife still in my hand. Covered in blood I was. I don't
remember a thing about it, but that's what they told me. At
the trial the prosecutor said the body was unrecognisable.

Murderess. My description in the newspaper. *A passionate
woman.* I liked that part. I didn't like the Italian professor.
He was a cold fish. He waited for me in the superintendent's
office and the warders took me up to him. He was doing
research, he said in his pompous Italian voice. Research into
the nature of the criminal mind. So he measured my head
and then had me undress and show him Jules's picture. As I
stood there half-naked he wrote things down and looked at
me, a hooded look which on the surface was supposed to
mean he thought I was nothing, and underneath meant just
the opposite. As they took me back out he was already
whispering to the superintendent, making his
arrangements, his request.

At my trial the magistrate condemned me to death. There
was no appeal. On the appointed morning I said my prayers
and was taken outside the prison gates, where there was a
large crowd waiting. Murderess! *Passionate woman.* The
noise was like the sea. They strapped me to the bascule of a
guillotine which had been brought out from Paris for the
express purpose of killing me. Imagine! The wind was
blowing and there was a taste of salt on the air.

Afterwards my body was the property of the state. At the
post-mortem examination they cut away the square of skin
over my heart and preserved it, as a demonstration of my
criminal nature. It was kept with many others, and that is

how it was bought by the collector, one of many anonymous
squares of skin, with on it a little picture of a man, a fine
man with a moustache wearing a striped jersey. All that was
left of me. Jules. My love.

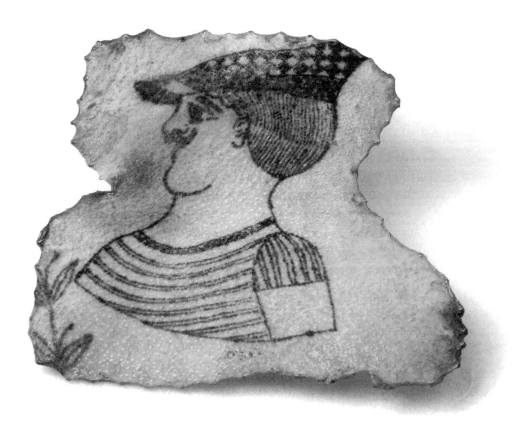

Even in nothingness one has to have something to think about.

I like to contemplate certain ironic aspects of my situation.
The one I like best is that the collector is here too, caught in
his own afterlife. Skin follicles. Saliva. A single moustache
hair that fell when he was examining a new curio. Enough to
trap him here, one of us, crouching in the darkness. So now
the millionaire, the gatherer of people and pieces of people
and pieces of people's lives, flits about amid the numberless
items in his collection like a very wealthy bat.

I enjoy that. It seems fitting.

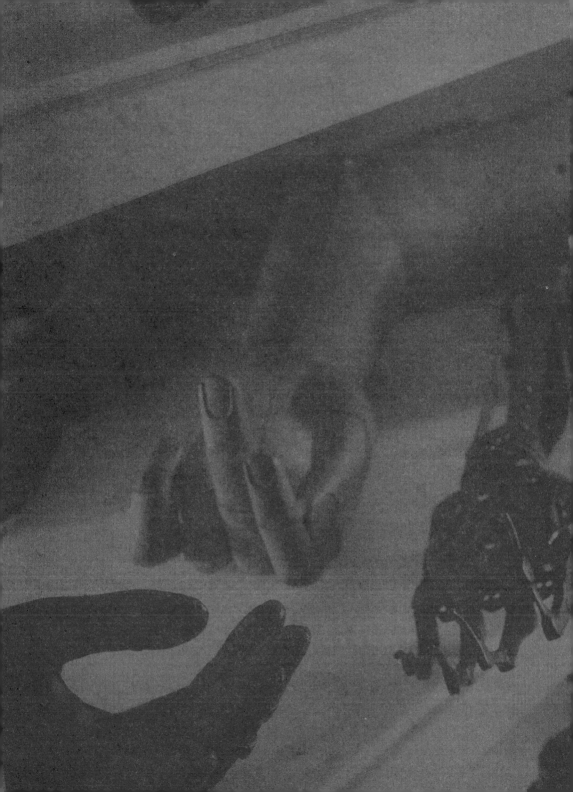

Gaby Wood
Phantom Limbs *or*
The Case of Captain Aubert
and the Bengal Tiger

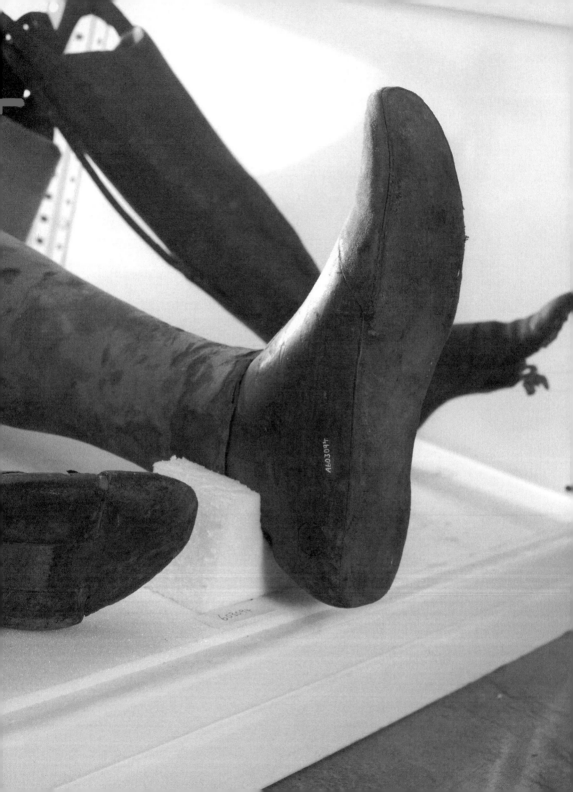

We regret much to have to record a sad accident which occurred in the Dhoon on the afternoon of the 16th instant. Captain Aubert, of the 34th N.I., Adjutant of Sumoor Battalion, having received information that a tiger had killed two bullocks and a man close to him, ordered out his elephant, and very soon reached the spot... The tiger immediately sprang on him, and seized him by one of his ankles; Captain Aubert succeeded at last in getting away with his ankle completely smashed, and actually walked towards a tree, and was attempting to get up it, when the tiger again rushed at him, seized his other leg with his claws, dragged him down, and again fastened on the wounded leg just below the knee... It may be understood in what a dreadful state Captain Aubert must have reached Dhera at about five o'clock in the morning of the 17th. One of his legs was immediately amputated above the knee; but the doctor is in hopes that, although dreadfully lacerated, the other may be saved, the patient bearing his sufferings with utmost fortitude.

The Delhi Gazette, 25 March 1848

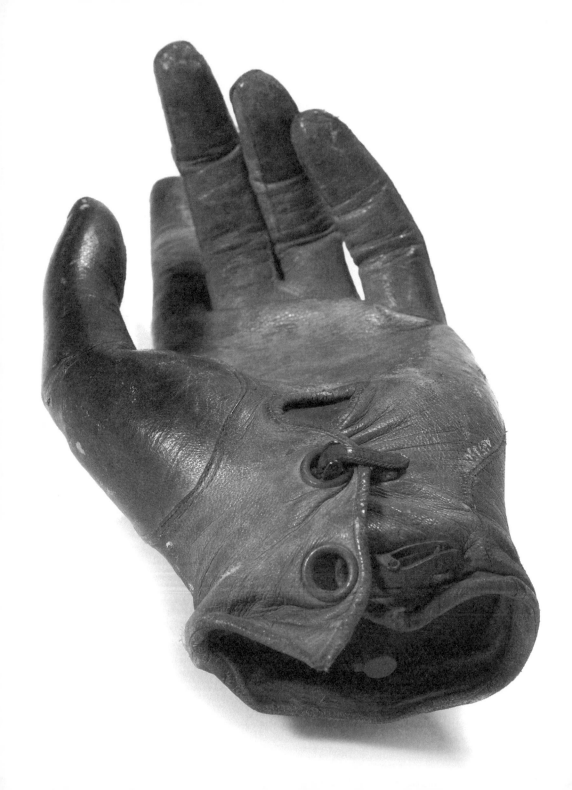

I N T H E S T O R E R O O M S O F T H E M U S E U M, stacked on shelves and arranged side by side like dolls laid to rest in a nursery, are parts of people. Brass legs laced up along the thigh, spidery steel-jointed arms, wooden hands wrapped in leather: not flesh or blood, but human remains nonetheless, remnants of their long-dead owners, clues to unknowable lives.

The legs lie stiff and unyielding, but the hands are caught in spasms of gesticulation. They seem to be pointing, or beckoning, fingers folding inwards – gesturing towards a story they cannot tell. Where have they been? What have they done? We know only, broadly, when they were made, and sometimes where. Yet each one must have changed or even saved a life: someone, to whom they were once attached, was robbed of a part of themselves, and then, given a simulacrum, could get dressed, return to work, eat, write or sew. Of these stories, these losses and rescues, we know nothing. The hands remain mute, frozen in a language of meaningless signs.

There is one, a delicate thing in a light-brown leather glove – perhaps a woman's. It was made in late nineteenth- or early twentieth-century Europe, and shows signs of wear – dark patches along the thumb muscle, heavy creases in the joints of each finger. There is something too intimate about it, perhaps because it looks so real, like any gloved hand; perhaps because of its polite gentility – the other hands on display are in a greater state of undress. This demure object seems to have more character than the rest: slain at the wrist, it offers itself up, palm towards the sky, pointing towards me two little clasps where, if it were living, an artery would be. In a moment of illicit curiosity I accept the apparent invitation, and undo the clasps.

As I slide the glove up over the smooth wooden wrist, the hand reveals more. Engraved into its surface, hidden beneath the leather, is a kind of message: two lines, like those read in palmistry. There is a head line, and a line for life, but there is no line for a heart.

Götz von Berlichingen, a sixteenth-century Bavarian knight and one of the earliest known owners of an artificial limb, was immortalised in a poem by Goethe, and given to say of his metal hand that it was 'insensible to the pressure of love'. The hand in the museum seems to say the same – that it has lost out on affairs of the heart – and something further, not about love but about life: that although its owner's heart was destined to stop, the hand had none and would never die. It would remain floating in the world, disembodied and senseless, a phantom of some former self.

*

In the mid-sixteenth century, the great French surgeon Ambroise Paré became the first to set down in writing a phenomenon he had observed among patients whose limbs he had amputated. As surgeon to the king, Paré accompanied Henri II on his campaigns against the English, and against the Holy Roman Emperor, Charles V. When mounting numbers of men were shot in battle, he altered his surgical procedures. Paré pioneered a new, safer method of amputation, and in the process he also discovered a strange fact: that men who had lost their limbs felt the limbs to be still there. Not only did the patients imagine them, but they sometimes felt pain in these limbs, tried to walk on their non-existent legs or reach for objects with a missing arm. Paré designed artificial body parts for his amputees, beautiful constructions to be made in metal by armourers, but he could do nothing for these strange configurations of the mind.

Centuries later, in the course of another war, the writer and neurologist Silas Weir Mitchell gave this phenomenon a name: he said his patients were suffering from 'phantom limbs' – since these 'vivid hallucinations' were in fact a form of haunting. 'Nearly every man who

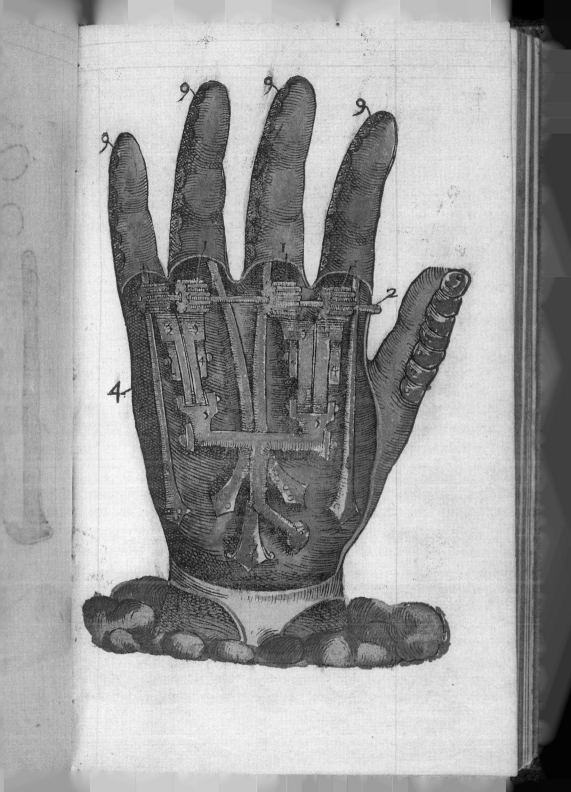

loses a limb,' Mitchell wrote, 'carries about with him a constant or inconstant phantom of the missing member, a sensory ghost of that much of himself.'

Mitchell was 33 years old when he became a contract surgeon for the Union Army during the American Civil War. His arrival at Gettysburg just after the famous battle made a deep impression on him, and ensured that he would despise conflict to the end of his days. There were 27,000 wounded to be cared for when he got there. Mitchell said he 'smelt nine hundred smells', and later spoke of 'the dead Confederates... with arms and legs in rigid extension – a most horrible memory'. He was eventually placed in charge of Turner's Lane Hospital in Philadelphia, which received a large number of nervous cases, and he made his reputation on the research he conducted into nerve injuries and gunshot wounds. He identified the condition that was to become known as shell shock, but was occupied more specifically with the thousands of amputees who populated the Philadelphia 'Stump Hospital'.

Writing in a popular magazine in 1871, Mitchell estimated that about 15,000 men across the country had lost an arm or a leg during the war, though only 6,075 of them had been supplied with artificial limbs so far. The sheer number of patients Mitchell saw allowed him to observe the 'strange and startling phenomena' associated with phantom limbs, a form of neuralgia he concluded must stem from inflamed or otherwise damaged nerves in the amputee's stump. Far from being an unusual condition, it was one Mitchell found to be present in all but five per cent of cases, and he could offer no explanation for the exceptions. He saw one man who was so sure of his missing arm that he went riding and used the lost hand to grasp the reins, causing an accident. Another thought he had punched someone, but realised he had taken aim with his phantom fist. A third complained of chronic nausea, since every time he sat down to eat he tried to pick up a fork and felt sick at his failure.

'There is something almost tragical, something ghastly,' Mitchell wrote, 'in the notion of these thousands of spirit limbs haunting as many good soldiers.' Indeed, in many cases he found a curious version of the commonly held belief about ghosts – that people who have died violently are condemned to roam the earth in the condition in which they have been left. Some amputees in Mitchell's care found their phantom limbs stuck in the position in which they had last felt them; the last real sensation in the limb remained forever, so that a phantom hand might be paralysed with the thumb cutting into the palm, or the fingers rigid in agony.

In the course of his article, Mitchell mentioned another, which had been published anonymously years earlier in the *Atlantic Monthly*. It was a 'humorous sketch', a 'jeu d'esprit', he said, whose fictional protagonist – a man who had lost all his limbs during the Civil War – was so believable that a number of readers had erroneously sent donations to him at the Stump Hospital. Mitchell portrayed this earlier article as an irresponsible piece of writing, and claimed that his own would describe, correctly and scientifically, the experiences of those haunted by phantom limbs.

As it happens, however, Mitchell was only correcting himself. 'The Case of George Dedlow', as the *Atlantic Monthly* story was called, was Mitchell's first attempt at writing fiction – a second career in which he was to excel. Far from being funny, it was a portrait of a man who had lost everything, including his sense of self, and it clearly succeeded in eliciting a good deal of sympathy from a general public who had until then believed, along with most doctors, that phantom limbs were all in the mind.

In the story, Dedlow describes himself as 'not a happy fraction of a man'. His arms are blown off, and later in the war he loses both legs: 'Against all chances I recovered, to find myself a useless torso.' He still feels his missing legs, however, and explains the medical reasons for this in layman's terms: the nerve, which once led to the extremity and remains in the stump, 'is like a bell-wire. You may pull it at any part of its course, and thus ring the bell as well as if you pulled at the end of the wire.'

Gradually, Dedlow experiences a psychic loss more dramatic than the physical loss of his limbs; as he lies in hospital, motionless and bed-bound, he feels his identity beginning to erode. He wonders 'how much a man might lose and yet live', since 'to lose any part must lessen his sense of his own existence'. Dedlow is so bewildered by his loss of self that he feels 'like

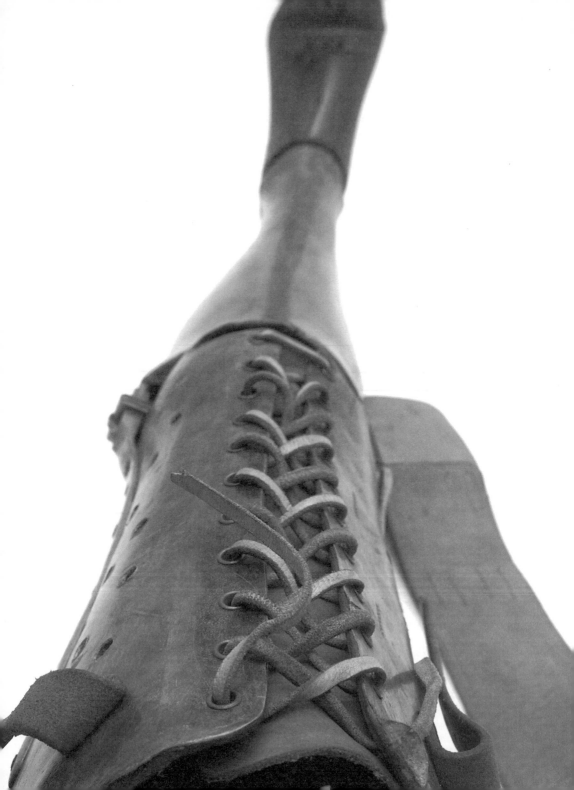

asking someone constantly if I were really George Dedlow or not... At times the conviction of my want of being myself was overwhelming and most painful.'

The story ends with a visit Dedlow makes to a spirit medium, who summons his amputated legs from the afterlife. They identify themselves – rapping on the table – by two numbers: their catalogue codes from the United States Army Medical Museum. Dedlow is, he says, 'reindividualized', returned to himself, and so entranced by this spirit communication that he walks across the room on invisible legs, astonishing everyone with his miraculous behaviour, before sinking feebly to the floor.

Mitchell's short story was an exaggeration, of course, but it encapsulated a number of things connected with phantom limbs, and by extension, with the artificial limbs designed to replace them. The limbs are called phantoms because they are felt manifestations of something that does not physically exist – they are, in Mitchell's words, 'sensory hallucinations'. But they are also phantoms in their connection to the spirit world – produced, like the ghosts of the dead, in response to a loss. No matter what the neurological explanation for the phenomenon, phantom limbs are a form of mourning – the body's, or the mind's, way of making up for what has gone. Whenever surgeons performed repeated amputations, shortening the stump incrementally in an attempt to rid the sufferer of his delusion, the phantom would return with a vengeance, reasserting itself with every loss. So much is the phantom limb connected to the notion of an afterlife that Lord Nelson, on losing his right arm in battle, believed the phantom arm that replaced it to be 'direct evidence for the existence of the soul'. If an arm could survive amputation, he proclaimed, why should an entire person not live on after death?

In a book entitled *The Phantom Limb Phenomenon* (1978), Douglas B. Price and Neil J. Twombly have collected a number of accounts, from the tenth century onwards, of the miraculous restoration of lost body parts, a common folkloric trope which they argue is related to the experience of phantom limbs. After all, is a person who believes his lost limb to have been restored to him by a miracle so different from the person who, sometimes weeks or years after the wound has healed, becomes conscious of his missing limb? Mitchell reported one case in which a patient had no phantom limb at all until two years after the amputation, when a mild electrical current was passed through his body, at which point he grasped at thin air and shouted in pain: 'Oh, the hand! The hand!' 'No resurrection of the dead, no answer of a summoned spirit, could have been more startling,' Mitchell wrote. Might the religious and medical narratives be analogous?

One of the miracle tales, so famous as to have been painted repeatedly (in one depiction by Fra Angelico), concerns a leg transplant performed by two saints, Cosmas and Damian. Summoned by Pope Felix to help a man whose leg is cancerous, Cosmas and Damian cut off the man's leg. But 'where,' they ask, 'shall we get flesh to fill up this void?' The angel Raphael appears to them and tells them that an Ethiopian has just been buried in a graveyard nearby. They are to dig up his body and cut off his leg. Then, the angel instructs them, on the day of the resurrection, they must orchestrate a swap. The saints do as they have been told, and sure enough, once the exchange has been effected, they see that each leg has become attached, by some miracle, to the person by whom they had lain it. The dead Moor has one white leg, and the man who had cancer awakes to find his leg fully functioning, though it is clearly, by its colour, someone else's.

'Putting then a candle nearby,' reads one account of this awakening, 'when he saw nothing wrong in the leg, he thought that he was not who he was, but someone else.' Another account, a poem in old English printed by William Caxton in 1483, reads as follows: 'and when the seke man a woke/ and felte no payne/ he put forthe his honde/ and felte his legge withoute hurte/ And thenne tooke a Candel/ and sawe wel that it was not his thye/ but that hit was a nother/ And when he was wel come to hym self/ he sprange oute of his bedde for joye.'

This story is not unlike that of George Dedlow needing to be reminded, as his physical self becomes more alien to him, that he is who he thinks he is. But unlike George Dedlow, this man does not recognise himself because he has acquired a body part that is foreign to him – something new has been

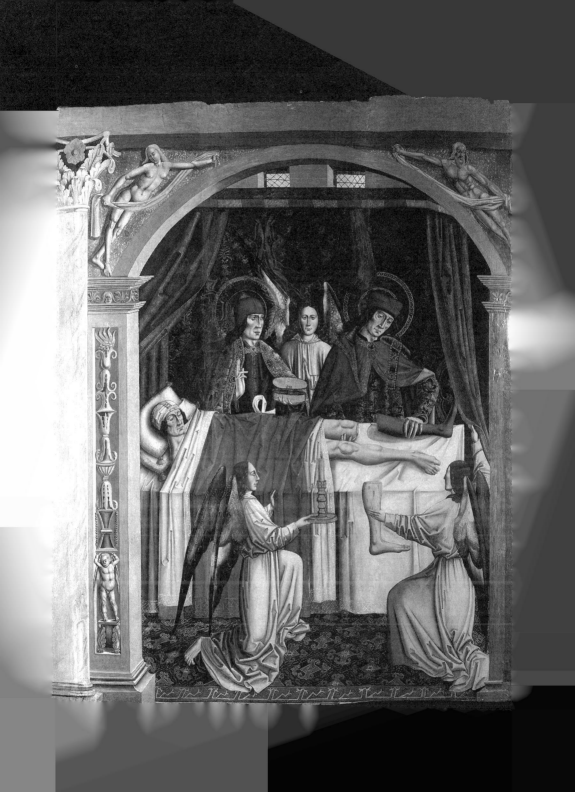

added. In that respect, he is more like a patient described by the contemporary neurologist Oliver Sacks. 'The man who fell out of bed', as Sacks calls him, suffers from a delusion that is a reversal of a phantom limb: he thinks his own leg is someone else's, stolen from the dissecting room and placed under the sheets of his hospital bed as a joke. But when he tries to throw the leg out of the bed the rest of his body goes with it, since it is in fact his own, and still attached. He ends up on the floor, and can't get up, because the leg he sees is so seemingly separate as to be of no use to him. He can't make it move because he is so disgusted by it that he is unable to accept it. He is horrified by the leg, calls it 'ghastly', 'uncanny', 'a counterfeit', and expresses some astonishment at the idea that anyone should have gone to such lengths as to manufacture 'a facsimile'.

In the story of the saintly transplant, it is no accident that the leg donor is a 'Moor'. The transplant is considered a miracle because the impossible has been performed: the donor was initially dead (so some form of resurrection is involved), and the knitting together of nerves, muscles and tissues required is so complex that surgeons are only now, in the 21st century, beginning to achieve success with such grafting of limbs. But part of the shock, for the patient and his acquaintances, is that the new, functioning body part should be so completely foreign to the white man. When he starts to walk around, no one who sees him believes the miracle until they go to the graveyard and see for themselves that the dead Ethiopian now possesses a white leg, that there has been a straight swap.

To the original readers of this story, there could be nothing more foreign than black skin to white. Taken metaphorically rather than literally, the scene is about one's sense of identity. The black leg might be alien for another reason – it might be wooden, or some other form of prosthetic, real or imagined. The story might not be about limbs at all, but about a state of mind – the splintering of the self. In the Caxton poem, the man has to wait a while before he is 'wel come to hym self': before he is fully awake perhaps, before he has 'well come' to his senses. But also, before he is welcome; like 'the man who fell out of bed', he cannot rise until he accepts who he is.

How many owners of artificial limbs have felt something like this when their prostheses were first delivered? How alien must they feel to themselves? What happens to phantom limbs when they are usurped by wooden or metal pretenders to their position?

While researching these issues, Oliver Sacks came across an interesting fact. Far from getting in the way of an artificial limb, a phantom turns out to be a prerequisite for wearing one. 'All amputees,' Sacks wrote in his book *The Man Who Mistook His Wife for a Hat*, 'and all who work with them, know that a phantom limb is essential if an artificial limb is to be used.' A fellow neurologist had written to Sacks that the phantom's 'value to the amputee is enormous. I am quite certain that no amputee with an artificial lower limb can walk on it satisfactorily until the body-image, in other words the phantom, is incorporated into it.' 'Thus,' Sacks concluded, 'the disappearance of a phantom may be disastrous, and its recovery, its reanimation, a matter of urgency. This may be effected in all sorts of ways... One such patient, under my care, describes how he must "wake up" his phantom in the mornings: first he flexes the thigh-stump towards him, and then he slaps it sharply – "like a baby's bottom" – several times. On the fifth or sixth slap the phantom suddenly shoots forth, rekindled, *fulgurated*, by the peripheral stimulus. Only then can he put on his prosthesis and walk.'

Another of Sacks's patients described the way in which his prosthetic limb helped with the pain in his phantom. 'There's this *thing*,' he said, 'this ghost-foot, which sometimes hurts like hell – and the toes curl up, or go into spasm. This is worst at night, or with the prosthesis off, or when I'm not doing anything. It goes away when I strap the prosthesis on and walk. I still feel the leg then, vividly, but it's a *good* phantom, different – it animates the prosthesis, and allows me to walk.'

The phantom, in other words, atrophies and causes pain without the prosthesis to give it purpose, and the prosthesis can only function when animated – literally given a soul, as Nelson would have it – by the phantom. The limb-wearer becomes a man-machine, given bionic life when 'fulgurated' or 'faradised', like the monster in Mary Shelley's *Frankenstein*.

The most recent research into phantom limbs, conducted by the American neurologist V. S. Ramachandran and popularised in his book

Phantoms in the Brain, shows that the phenomenon may be connected to a sort of 'artificial man' in the human brain. There is, on the brain's surface, a map of the body in the awkward shape of a man. The map is known as 'the Penfield homunculus'. In the homunculus, the hand and thumb are next to the face. When Ramachandran experimented with a phantom-hand patient by lightly rubbing his cheek, the patient confirmed that he felt the rubbing in his missing hand. In other words, in cases of phantom limbs, the brain receives messages in a neighbouring area, though that area is not, on the external human body, adjacent. Other patients confirmed this theory. For example, two people reported sensations in their phantom foot when they had sex, and were astonished to discover an explanation for this: in the brain, on the Penfield map, the genitals and the feet are next to each other. 'I never suspected,' Ramachandran wryly concludes, 'that I would begin seeking an explanation for phantom limbs and end up explaining foot fetishes as well.'

But Ramachandran also wanted to help his patients who had pain in their phantoms, or found them paralysed, as Mitchell's patients had, in the position in which they'd last felt them. He developed a novel technique for this, which involved giving the patient the impression that the phantom they felt but could not see was physically present. He constructed a 'virtual reality box', with a vertical mirror inside it and two holes in the front. He asked patients to put both arms through the holes and to move them about in tandem. With the help of the mirror in reversing the arms, the patients saw their phantoms actually move. In some cases the paralysis ended; in others the phantoms disappeared altogether, along with the pain. What appeared to have been performed, as Ramachandran put it, was 'the first example in medical history of a successful "amputation" of a phantom limb'. 'Philip,' he said of one of his patients, 'seemed to think I was some kind of magician'; and indeed the 'virtual reality box' he invented is not unlike the cabinet tricks used by stage magicians in the nineteenth century. The doctor had cured a delusion using illusionism.

In fact there are many ways in which the history of artificial limbs overlaps with that of various forms of magic. There is the uncanny aspect –

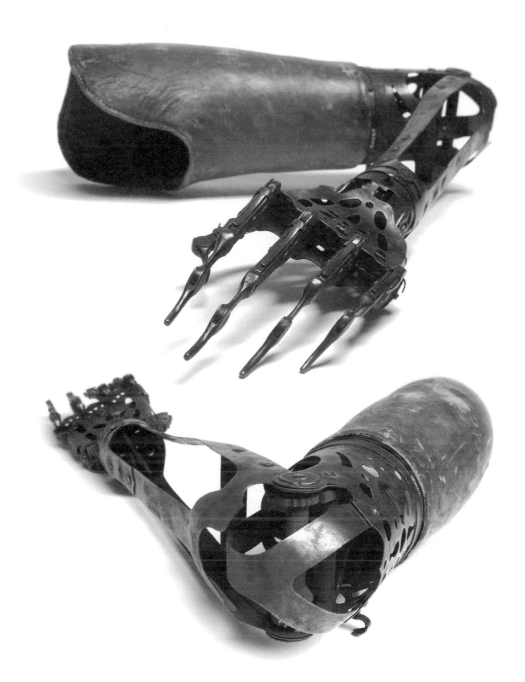

the apparent bringing forth of ghosts – and there is a technical side as well. In a number of cases, mechanicians who made artificial beings intended for entertainment – androids or automata – also developed technology used in prosthetics.

One famous instance of this is the mechanical Turk, also known as the Automaton Chess Player, built in 1769 by a Hungarian civil servant named Wolfgang von Kempelen. The Turk, who was dressed in the obscure attire of the East (a wilful effect of foreignness reminiscent of the miraculous Moor) was a kind of puppet that played chess. There seemed to be no human operating force inside the large cabinet at which it sat and played, and for decades audiences all over Europe and America believed it to be a genuine artificial intelligence machine. But there was, in fact, a hidden player – who won every game through the medium of the figure's artificial arm, picking up chess pieces and releasing them using a set of levers and cranks. In this sense, the entire 'automaton' was a kind of prosthesis for the human chess player, who was never allowed to be seen, his identity given over to that of his more famous inanimate counterpart.

But who exactly was animating whom? When the philosopher Walter Benjamin wrote about the Turk he spoke of the way in which it 'enlist[ed] the services' of the man inside it – in other words, the puppeteer was in the service of the puppet. In this view of the automaton, the machine called the shots, and the man was entirely subject to it. In a practical sense, the Turk eventually helped humans: the chess-playing arm was a sophisticated piece of mechanism, whose design contributed to the future manufacture of artificial limbs. Yet the problem of what one observer called 'the Siamese relationship of body and board' remained. Was there a ghost in the machine, or was the machine itself the only phantom, teasing audiences with its invisible life-force and unfathomable existence? Like Oliver Sacks's patient, the real man and his artificial extension needed each other in order to survive.

*

For centuries, the history of prosthetics has been the history of war. The earliest written account of an artificial limb is in Sanskrit. It appears in the holy Indian text, the Rig-Veda, written between 3500 and 1800 BC, and tells the story of a warrior queen named Vishpla, who lost her leg in battle, and, when fitted with an iron prosthesis, returned to the scene of the fighting.

In 1508, Götz von Berlichingen, then a 23-year-old knight, lost his right arm during the siege of Landshut. The iron limb subsequently made for him by his armourer became the feature by which this valiant protector of the people could be most easily identified. In Goethe's poem about him, a monk who asks him to introduce himself becomes offended when the knight extends his left hand rather than his right. But when he sees that the right is made of metal, the monk no longer needs an introduction. Götz's fame precedes him; the monk falls to his knees and kisses the prosthesis as a mark of his admiration. In fact, Götz said that his artificial hand made him a better warrior, made him superhuman in a way. 'It has rendered more service in the fight,' he said of his prosthesis, 'than ever did the original of flesh.'

Not long afterwards, Ambroise Paré made substantial improvements to such pieces of human armour; he designed a whole arm, jointed at the elbow, an adjustable metal leg and a hand operated by springs which was made for a captain in the French Army and became known as 'Le Petit Lorrain'.

With each great conflict came new weapons and new casualties; medical supplies improved, technology progressed, compensation arrangements changed. The Battle of Waterloo, the American Civil War, World Wars One and Two all mark turning points in the advance of artificial limbs.

One legendary owner of an artificial leg was Lord Uxbridge, later to become the Marquess of Anglesey. The man was second-in-command to the Duke of Wellington, and known for his military achievements, but the leg became famous mainly because of the bathos with which it was lost. As Uxbridge and Wellington rode out side by side across the fields of the Battle of Waterloo, Wellington proudly surveying his victory, Uxbridge's

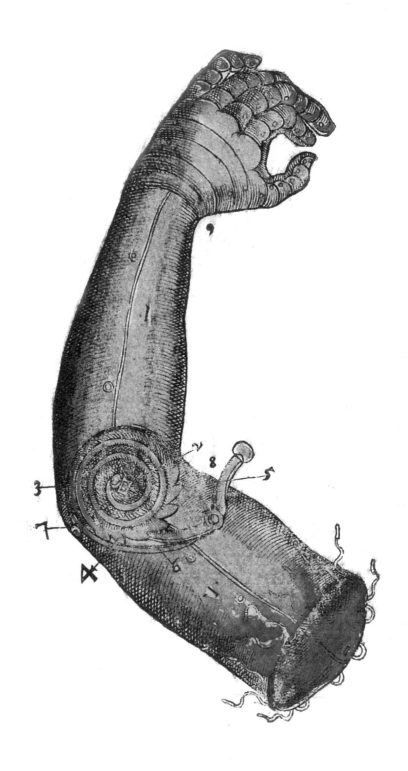

leg was blown off by the last shot fired. 'By God, sir,' he said to his riding companion, 'I've lost my leg!' Wellington took his eye from his telescope for a moment, looked down and said, 'By God, sir, so you have!' He then returned to his view of the landscape.

The Marquess of Anglesey had an artificial leg made by a man named James Potts, whose own loss of limb had led him to design them, and this became known as the 'Anglesey Leg'. It was made in 1815, and exported to the United States 24 years later. The Marquess's real leg, meanwhile, continued a 'phantom' existence of its own peculiar kind. In the garden of the house in Belgium where it was amputated, there remains to this day a monument to the shattered limb.

The American Civil War saw unprecedented numbers of men made limbless; Silas Weir Mitchell's early estimate of 15,000 turned out to be conservative – there were around twice that many amputations conducted in the Union Army. The poet Walt Whitman worked in a field hospital as a volunteer nurse, and saw on his arrival the remains of countless operations. There was, he wrote, 'a heap of feet, legs, arms and human fragments, a full load for a one-horse cart'. But surgery was safer and less painful than it had been before – ether and chloroform were now used, and the longer operating time these allowed made for more effective stumps. In 1862, a year after the war began, the United States government provided funding for one free prosthesis per amputation for soldiers and sailors, and the spread of the Industrial Revolution meant that these devices could be greatly improved.

Whilst the Civil War marked a turning point in the history of American prosthetics, there was no change on this scale in Europe until the First World War. The year before war broke out, there were only 34 amputations performed at St Thomas's Hospital in London, out of a total of 5,483 major operations. By 1918, His Majesty's Ministry of Pensions was faced with the problem of rehabilitating over 40,000 limbless ex-Service men. In 1915, Queen Mary's Convalescent Military Hospital was founded in Roehampton in South London to care exclusively for men who had lost their limbs. Artificial limbs were made on site by J. E. Hanger and

Company, the largest artificial limb works in the world, with 400 skilled craftsmen in constant employment.

During the war, a set of practical treatises was published as part of a series called Oxford War Primers, and during the Second World War they were revised. The Rt Hon. Lord Horder, general editor of the series, prefaced the 1944 edition of *Amputations and Artificial Limbs* with these stirring words: 'If any good is to emerge from the evil which confronts us today, it will be salvaged in the form of medical progress accelerated through intensity of experience.' As it happened, the medical lessons learned in the previous war had a pronounced effect on the second. In 1939, Queen Mary's Hospital expanded their limb fitting centre and factory, in memory of the 40,000 limb casualties of the last war and in anticipation of large numbers still to come. But there were approximately half the number of amputees during the Second World War, a fact Leon Gillis, Consultant Surgeon at QMH and an expert on artificial limbs, ascribed to 'advances in surgical techniques, in chemotherapy and in the general management of any injury, better treatment of infection and the availability of blood transfusion'.

War was not the only cause of limb loss: mass production meant that workers suffered accidents in factories; the advent of the railways in the nineteenth century caused further accidents, as did traffic with the widespread use of cars. Nevertheless, this is a broad sort of history, a political or industrial history. It gives a sense of the general sweep of things, but it brings us no closer to the individuals who lost parts of themselves. During all the wartime advances, for instance, not a single prosthetic leg in any one of the advertisements or pamphlets was designed for a woman. The casualties in this history were all men, and yet we know that women lost hands, arms and legs – in accidents, or to disease. How can we get closer to the personal history, the experience of such loss or recovery of one's self, to the thoughts, lives or names of the people who once animated the objects in our museum?

*

One way might be through the manufacturers themselves. In 1945, the American National Academy of Sciences established their first Artificial Limb Program, because they had stumbled across a curious fact. No concerted effort had ever been made to conduct research into artificial limbs, they found; those that existed had all been invented by men like James Potts, who, in the words of the man who was to take over his business, had 'unfortunately for himself, but as it eventually proved, fortunately for others, lost a leg'. These people had designed prostheses for themselves, and then gone on to make their inventions available commercially. For the Academy of Sciences, this meant there was a good deal of medical and engineering research to be done. But it also meant that for every limb, there was a story...

A brochure published in the 1910s by the Carnes Artificial Limb Company of Kansas City claimed that 'any one finger of our Hands will carry 25 pounds without straining it in the least'. The Carnes hands were made of hard, vulcanised fibre, the sockets of willow and the mechanical parts of cold rolled steel. An order form was inserted at the back of the brochure, with directions for measuring, and for taking plaster of Paris casts of the stump. Clients were asked to 'send a glove for the artificial hand'.

The front of the brochure was taken up with the story of how the Carnes Arm came into being. Under the heading 'Necessity is the Mother of Invention' is the true story of William T. Carnes.

> On the night of 13th February 1902, William T. Carnes, a machinist of Warren, Pennsylvania, was working on a large boring and milling machine in a machine shop at Pittsburgh, when his right arm came in contact with a revolving cog-wheel and was so terribly lacerated that it was necessary for it be amputated two inches above the elbow.
>
> After leaving the hospital, Mr Carnes endeavored to get something in the artificial line that would allow him to continue at his trade. With this thought he visited a number of artificial limb factories to learn just what there was on the market, and this fact he discovered – that artificial arms were more ornamental than useful, and very little of either.

After wearing for a short time an arm which he purchased of a firm in Pittsburgh, he started to build one for himself. He studied very carefully the anatomy of the human arm and fingers and combined their natural principles in an arrangement of steel levers, ratchet gearing and cranks in such a way that they would readily respond to the muscle force and the nerve impulses of the stump to which the arm is attached and, at the will of the operator, the arm is flexed or straightened, and the fingers open and close in a natural manner, enabling the wearer to carry a weight of 50 pounds with ease.

Never before, probably, had a man lost his own arm who had the mechanical skill, the patience and perseverance to work out each individual movement and test and try it out personally, patiently and painstakingly, changing this, condemning that, adapting a piece of mechanism only after thoroughly proving its superiority, completing one movement before working on the next one, finishing it, making them work in unison easily and naturally; strengthening the weak parts, hardening the wearing surfaces, etc, until in the face of untold discouragement, adverse criticism and friendly advice to 'drop it', he perfected the arm we now offer to the unfortunate as the BEST SUBSTITUTE for the natural arm ever invented.

To build this first arm was a great and tedious labor, as it was necessary to perform all the work with one hand; but since its completion he has been able to use the artificial member with great skill in the manufacture of other arms, thus demonstrating the wonderful success of his invention.

Still, William Carnes would have been making artificial arms in small numbers had another 'unfortunate' not come along. And so the brochure continued with the story of Mr J. P. Prescott, President and Treasurer of the company, who, on 16 December 1908, was caught in the freight elevator of his warehouse, suffering the loss of his left arm and right leg. He heard about the Carnes arm and went to have one fitted. When he arrived at the workshop,

He found Mr Carnes turning out arms so slowly that people who earnestly desired to secure them simply had to wait their turns. 'You really haven't a moral right to keep people waiting months for your arms,' he told Mr Carnes.

Prescott, who had experience in the railroads and the milling business, offered to set up a company for Carnes, and within two years Carnes arms were worn in 32 states and in Canada. Not only had the business been set up by two people who had lost their limbs, but all of their travelling salesmen were amputees and wearers of the arm as well. 'You do not have to rely upon their assertions,' the brochure boasted, 'but can see for yourself when one of our men calls upon you'.

Eleven years after William Carnes lost his arm at the factory, an Englishman lost a leg in a flying accident. A slim volume, published in 1922 and ambiguously titled *Progress*, recounts the story of this legacy of invention. Shortly after Blériot flew across the English Channel, the young Marcel Desoutter took up aeronautical engineering, and taught himself to fly. He met with some success as an aviator until, on a trip in 1913, he shattered his left leg, which was amputated when tetanus set in, leaving eight inches of stump.

Desoutter tried an artificial limb made in the United States, then French and British brands, but his primary aim was to return to the air, and all the prostheses available were far too heavy. Using a lightweight metal alloy that had only recently been developed – a form of aluminium used by the Wright brothers in the construction of their first plane – Marcel and his brother Charles (also an aeronautical engineer) designed a new leg. They were 'ridiculed by other limb-makers' at first, but within a year, Marcel was in a plane again.

'Mr Desoutter is, as far as can be ascertained, the only man to have flown an aeroplane whilst wearing an artificial leg for an amputation above the knee,' the book proclaimed, opposite a photograph of Marcel looking heroic in a monoplane. There he is, beret swept back over his head, goggles hovering over a thick black moustache. 'We would like to point out to the uninitiated,' the caption quibbled, 'that to fly the old Blériot monoplane necessitated a large amount of rudder-bar work, which was controlled by the legs. Only the efficiency of the "Desoutter" light-metal leg made this possible.'

A quote from the *Sunday Times* of 3 May 1914 was printed beneath this.

Marcel Desoutter, who had the misfortune to lose a leg as a result of an aeroplane accident, made a dramatic appearance at Hendon recently, when he landed with a 50 h.p. Blériot which he had piloted from Weybridge. Desoutter was quite delighted, as it is the desire of his life to be flying again.

Soon enough, however, the Desoutter brothers yielded to the desire of other people's lives, and Marcel gave up flying in order to manufacture the 'Desoutter leg' in large numbers. They were, it was advertised, 'perfectly natural in appearance'; 'cool, healthy, no perspiration'. An above-knee amputation leg took three to six weeks and five fittings to make, and cost 80 guineas. The 'Desoutter' heavily influenced the legs manufactured by J. E. Hanger at Roehampton Hospital during the First World War.

What of the hundreds who wore these limbs? Not the inventors or heroes, but the ordinary men and women, the clients?

Reproduced in the Carnes brochure are photographs of satisfied customers, along with, in many cases, thank-you letters written with the aid of the artificial arm in question. The company slogan was 'The Carnes Arm Puts You on the Pay Roll', and work was precisely the issue at stake. It was all very well if you were the Marquess of Anglesey, or had the entrepreneurial zeal of Marcel Desoutter, but in general, how would the limbless earn a living without decent prostheses? Would they even, in other words, survive at all? The Carnes success stories included Mr Wetmiller, a butcher, seen sharpening knives and cutting meat; Mr Lynch, a pool hall proprietor, cue poised over a pool table; Mr Harrington, a bookkeeper, doing deals on the phone, mouthpiece in one hand, earpiece in the other. There was Mr Hobson, who sent pictures of himself playing the violin and riding a bike, and a grateful Miss Gladys Bradley, shown at her domestic labours – sewing, ironing and sweeping at last.

An earlier limb-maker, Frederick Gray, who continued the work of James Potts in London, had clients so well known he felt it inappropriate, in many cases, to mention them by name. But he too had something important to say about less wealthy limb-wearers. 'Before I proceed to transcribe some of the cases in which my mode of supplying artificial limbs has been eminently successful,' Gray wrote in 1855, 'I will state my regret that, from the expense entailed by their elaborate construction, they are not within the reach of the poorer class of sufferers. This is the more to be regretted, because in the case of the affluent the loss of a limb does not reduce the sufferer to a state in which his relative position in life is rendered worse, whereas, when a poor man becomes crippled, he is reduced to a state of almost perfect destitution and misery.' In a footnote added later, Gray mentioned that one of his wealthier clients had, on his recommendation, established an association with the aim of 'furnishing artificial limbs to the poor, both military and civil'.

For each case, Gray gave an account of the artificial limb's making: he recorded whether the patient was 'stout' or 'spare' (affecting the weight put on the prosthesis), who performed the amputation, what type of surgery was involved, and a sense of the new limb's success. He listed, clearly desperate to give as many clues to their distinguished identities as he could: 'a clergyman, a near-relative to a late bishop of great eminence'; 'Prince G., a Russian general who lost his leg in the service of the Czar'; 'Master E., the 8-year-old son of an English lord'; 'the stout son of a late Baronet'. And then, a strange, floating mystery: 'Case XCIX, Mrs... This lady was one of the victims of the horrible tragedy enacted a few years ago in Norfolk, the perpetrator of which expiated his crime on the scaffold.'

The anonymous lady was not the only one whose loss of limb told a potentially gripping story. One of Gray's patients was at the centre of an imperial tragedy so striking that, though he mentioned him only by his initial, Gray permitted himself to reprint an article about the incident from the *Delhi Gazette* of 25 March 1848. We know from the newspaper clipping that the man's name was Captain Aubert, and that he was nearly the victim of an unfortunate family fate. Aubert's father and brother had both been killed, on separate occasions, when they fell from their horses, and another brother had died after being struck down by lightning. Though his leg was ripped off by a tiger, Aubert, it seemed, was lucky to be alive. The story takes place in the Bengali jungle, and in Frederick Gray's telling, it goes like this:

> The elephant upon which he was mounted, being a young one, became alarmed at the roaring of the tiger, and rushed beneath a tree. Captain A..., to prevent having his back broken by the branches, caught hold of one of them, and remained suspended by his hands and arms thereto for some time; the elephant meanwhile escaped. Immediately beneath the captain lay the tiger, which had been wounded by a ball. The captain's strength failing him, he at length fell, and the tiger seized upon him, lacerating his legs in so dreadful a manner, that one of them was obliged to be amputated above the knee... The captain is now about 36 years of age; he is moderately stout. He wore the common wooden leg, and suffered much from pressure... He has for some time worn my invention, and his health and energy are perfectly restored. He can ride and walk with comfort and ease, and so completely is the loss of his limb supplied by my contrivance, that he is about to return to India to resume his military duties.

*

What is the moral of this story? Is a return to the scene of the accident really the best thing that could have happened to Captain Aubert? Clearly, from Frederick Gray's point of view, this is a happy ending. Aubert is a hero, patriotically resuming the military duties that led to his unfortunate loss in the first place, defending the British Empire against the risks of the alien East. The story reads something like a fairy tale – 'The Case of

Captain Aubert and the Bengal Tiger', perhaps.

In her classic book on the genre, *From the Beast to the Blonde*, Marina Warner described the conclusions of fairy tales not as bringing about 'total closure' but as giving us a picture of the heroes going back to their ordinary lives. There is something open-ended, even unsettling, about them. We might wish for 'happily ever after', but the truth is, we don't know what will be. 'The genre,' Warner writes, 'is characterised by "heroic optimism", as if to say, "one day, we might be happy, even if it won't last".'

Fairy tales, Warner says, are also characterised by metamorphosis – limbs can be cut off and restored overnight, just the sort of magic trick that reports of miracles attributed to religion. People are made strange to themselves, and made whole again. These are acts of horror and acts of wonder rolled into one. Nightmares, fairy tales, epiphanies, tragedies and neurological disorders all share strikingly similar narratives; they are phantoms of the mind.

And since fairy tales can often serve the purpose of parables or foundation myths, The Case of Captain Aubert and the Bengal Tiger might be seen to stand for other stories still undocumented, might help us to reattach the memory of a person to each phantom in the museum. How else, after all, are we to make sense of these bodies in pieces? How many limbs, worn without fanfare and left behind after their owner's death, might lead backwards to silent voices, salvaged lives?

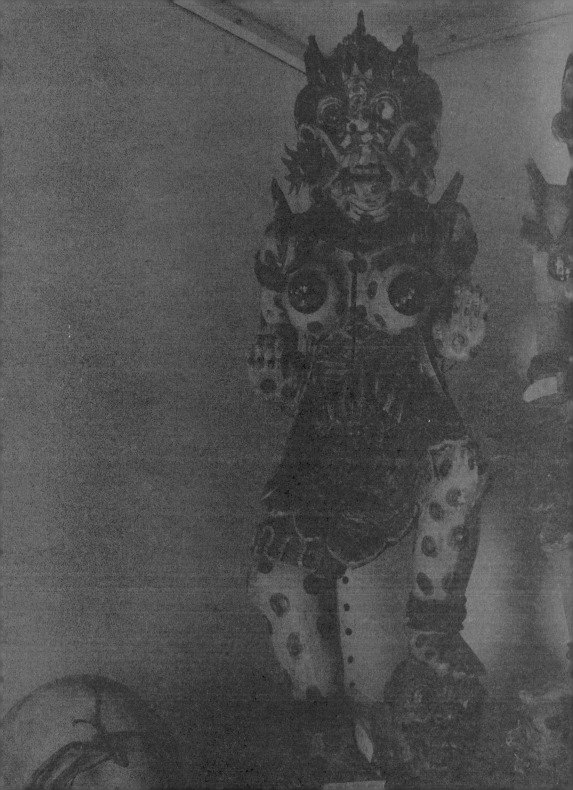

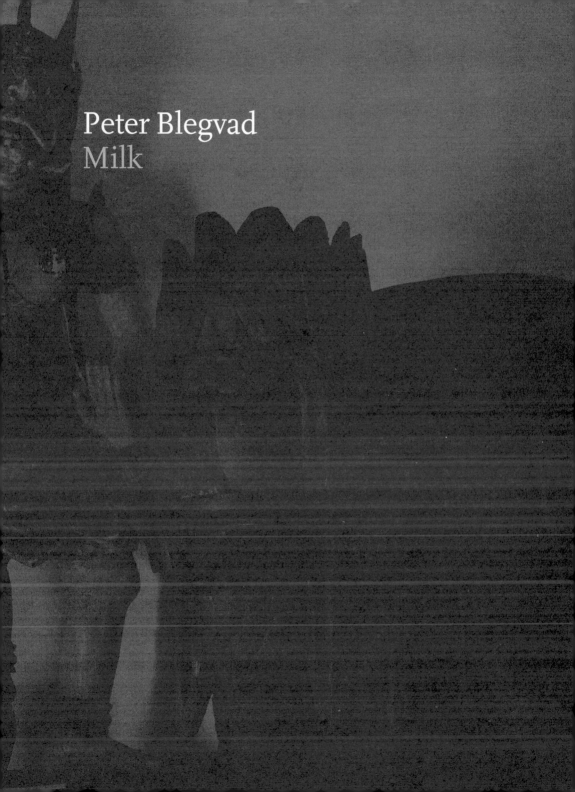

Peter Blegvad
Milk

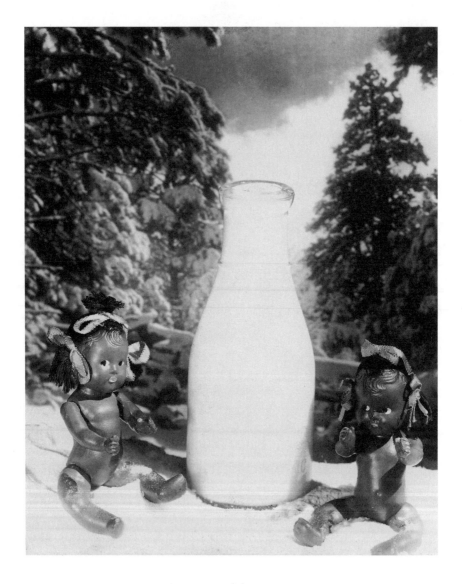

ADVERTISEMENT FOR MILK(?) PROVENANCE UNKNOWN
From a NYC flea market

MILK

MATTER OF LIFE AND DEATH

AN EXHIBITION OF RARE AND CURIOUS OBJECTS
FROM THE COLLECTION OF SIR HENRY WELLCOME
ORGANISED BY, AND UNDER THE DIRECTION OF
PETER BLEGVAD
ASSISTED BY
HILDI HAWKINS AND DANIELLE OLSEN

MILK:
AN IMMERSION FOR THIRSTY MINDS

The human mind is often stirred by what might be called the encyclopedic urge, the thirst to know everything. There are two approaches one can take to quench this thirst:

1.   The horizontal – learning a little about a lot of things.
2.   The vertical – learning a lot about one thing.

For many years I have taken the latter course, immersing myself in milk, acquiring a bale of quotes and a morgue of pictures pertaining to the stuff in order to test the theory that a sufficiently obsessive study of one thing will eventually result in a complete education about everything. There are two approaches one can take to research:

1.   The active – deliberately looking a subject up in reference works, typing it into search engines, etc.
2.   The passive – stumbling on a reference to the subject purely by chance, in the course of one's general reading, say, or hearing it mentioned in a song, a movie, a conversation, a dream, etc.

For many years I opted for the latter, acquiring information and images about milk serendipitously rather than by design. This guaranteed that finds were rare enough to seem oracular. Passive research is less work than play, it's the method of the amateur, guaranteed to produce happy and inexplicable results. It feeds obsession. But over the years I've grown increasingly curious to know what active research, a more professional approach, might yield. So last year, when Danielle Olsen and Hildi Hawkins invited me to interrogate the objects in Henry Wellcome's collection and to organise an exhibition of them, I recognised that the time had come to take the plunge.

For me that phrase, 'take the plunge', evokes immersion. It also evokes initiation, a ritualised enactment of death followed by rebirth. Before I took the plunge, my condition was one of incoherence, I was like

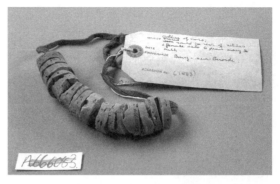

unto a haphazard collection of disparate things without a unifying narrative. One day I shall emerge from the milk made whole, making sense. With that goal in mind I typed MILK into the search engines of the Wellcome Library and the Science Museum. The ground shook, the earth swelled, a geyser gushed forth of matters lactic!

The tag tells us this (above) is a 'bootlace threaded with corks', and that it was 'placed around the necks of female cats or bitches to drain away their milk'. Where? 'Boring-sur-Gironde, France'. When? '1871–1920'. That's enough to be going on. To get the imagination going.

We're told what, where, when. Not why. Why might someone want to drain the milk from a cat or dog? Don't know? Good. Savour your freedom to speculate. My lazy first guess was that starving an unwanted litter to death saved someone the trouble of dispatching them. I drew the unhappy

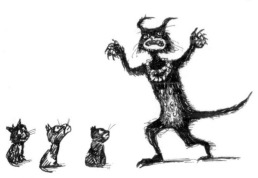

mother cat wailing to her kits that her milk has drained away (left). Realising this was ridiculous, I began to interrogate the object in verses which I wrote on tags (overleaf) to be tied to the amulet as an amateur alternative to professional museum labelling.

Interrogating an Amulet

1. A bootlace strung with bungs of cork
Was hung around a female cat
or bitch's neck to drain its milk.
What magic logic made it work?

In the photograph it's hard
to read the writing on the card
which might locate the loop of lace.

2. Is there really such a place
as BORING-sur-Gironde?
Autre temps, un autre monde,
1871 - 1920.
Sense of plethora, of plenty
latent in a lanyard which
once collared farmyard cat or bitch.

3. When fact is crossed with fantasy
we call the product history.
Good luck to he or she defends
where one starts and the other ends

4. Was cork naïvely thought to plug
the dugs the way it stops a jug?
And why might someone way back then
consider that a dividend?

Was it to deny supply
to someone with the evil eye?
Was the milk of beasts like these
sought for voodoo recipes,

5. pinched in darkness by a witch
from nipples of a cat or bitch?
Used in spells intending harm
to the souls who worked the farm?
Or, a surplus litter drowned,
would farmer tie this charm around
the mother's neck to make ammends
hoping they could still be friends?

6. Compassionate, in sympathy,
ADMINISTERED as therapy,
to nurse a swollen, pek distressed,
who writhed with matter unexpressed,
whose progeny was not on hand
or mouth to drain the angry gland.
Quell.

HISTORICAL MILK EXHIBITION

Sir Henry Wellcome (1853–1936) intended his collection to be a history of the evolution of medicine told in objects. From womb to tomb, flesh is heir to a multitude of afflictions, each with its own history of treatments involving objects of some kind. By 1931 his collection was five times larger than the Louvre's, but for all his wealth and ambition he died before he could organise it into anything like a coherent narrative. After his death the body of materials he'd spent so long and so much amassing was broken up, subjected to a sparagmos, dispersed.

Collecting is easy, connecting is hard. As a life-long collector myself, I know what it's like to be in the grip of the compulsion to add to a hoard which is already too big to house or make sense of.

The emblem on the Exhibition T-shirt (right) sums up the collector's lot. The Latin translates as 'My very plenty makes me poor.' Collectors, even wealthy ones, will understand.

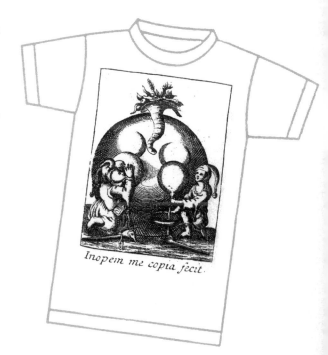

Inopem me copia fecit.

The Milk Exhibition is a history of human development from conception to corruption told in objects pertaining to milk. The biological name for our class of animal, Mammalia, is derived from the gland which gives milk. On land, the first act of the newborn mammal is to draw breath. But the next is to seek the mammary gland. Ostensibly, we're weaned of our dependency on milk early on. The Milk Exhibition suggests, on the contrary, that the oral fixations we graduate to – rubber teats and dummies, solid foods, alcohol, drugs, sex,[1] speech – are all surrogates for the suckling function which continues to haunt our largely unacknowledged reveries[2] until the earth, the Great Mother, takes us back to Her bosom. Milk resonates as a symbol of regression, arrested development, morbid dependency. It becomes the paradigm for all the habits we must kick if we're to progress.

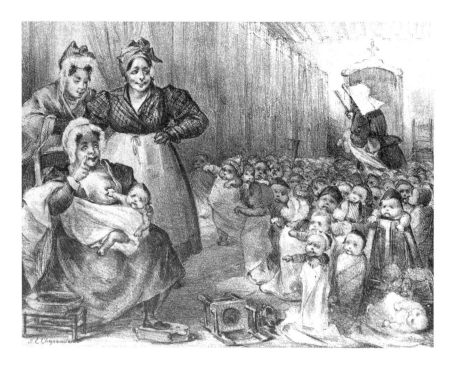

<u>Zombie Tots</u>

A sea of tots arrives in waves
summoned from their tiny graves.
Zombie babies in a trance
are made to do a clumsy dance.
Arms out like somnambulists,
their chubby fingers forming fists,
they slip, they trip, they catch their feet
on mummy-cloth and winding-sheet.

---

1 'It seems not only that the adult male becomes in face-to-face copulation, a surrogate suckling to the adult female by virtue of his position; but also that the adult female becomes a surrogate suckling to the male by virtue of her behaviour, which is that of soliciting and receiving a life-giving liquid from an adult bodily protuberance.' Wescott 1968, 92, quoted in *Bononbo the Forgotten Ape*, by Frans de Waal, University of California Press, 1997

2 'The insight of Freudian psychiatry that pictures many adults as subconsciously seeking the pleasant mouth satisfactions they felt as infant breast feeders and as small children opened up vistas for the depth merchandisers.' 'Motivational analysts turned their attention, in particular, to the hidden meanings of milk, milk products, liquids in general, and the softer foods. Social Research, for example, made a thorough study of the hidden satisfactions obtained from milk and found considerable documentation that milk is indeed psychically loaded. The experience of the military during the Second World War was cited in particular. It seems that soldiers who had been tried beyond their limit in combat and developed gastro-intestinal symptoms frequently revealed a common trait: a craving for milk.' Vance Packard, 'Back to the Breast and Beyond', *The Hidden Persuaders*, David McKay, 1957

Wellcome's collection is brimming with milk. More than 700 milk-related items – books, pamphlets, articles, objects, pictures – were churned up by the search engine in the Wellcome Library. These were divided into such categories as Milk – chemistry; Milk Ejection; Milk fever in animals; Milk, Human; Milk Hypersensitivity; Milk plants; Milk – radiation effects; Milk – toxicity; Milk – urine; Milking machines; Milk – therapeutic use; Milk Cakelettes; Milk of Roses; Milky Way... the list goes on for several pages. Given such a plethora, will active research exhaust my interest in the subject? Will the plunge prove purgative? Will it cure me? I'm sick of milk. I want to be weaned. While primarily a discourse with myself, I hope the Milk Exhibition may be of benefit to others who, like me, seek a second birth, initiation. Who want to fly out of the 'sorrowful weary wheel' of obsessive fixation.

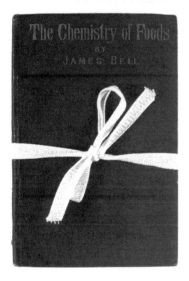
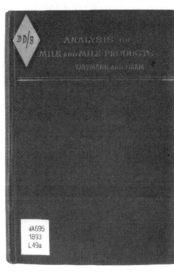
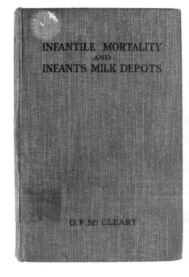

A GUIDED TOUR OF
THE MILK EXHIBITION

Above the entrance to the Milk Exhibition are two Walter Benjamin quotes:

"I needn't say anything. Merely show."

"Ideas are to objects as constellations are to stars."

THE FIRST ROOM

In the first room, once our eyes have adjusted to the gloom, we discover a constellation of dozens of glowing items. What unites them is the theme of immersion, of 'taking the plunge' into milk. Each item is linked to others by a maze of drawn lines or laser beams indicating vectors of correspondence. The initial impression of labyrinthine confusion is not accidental. The exhibition is designed to disorientate the viewer in the way that neophytes were disorientated preparatory to rebirth rituals. Rather than making the relationship between the exhibits explicit and drawing specific conclusions therefrom, the viewer is invited to exercise the faculty which Keats called 'Negative Capability, that is when man is capable of being in uncertainties, Mysteries, doubts, without any irritable reaching after fact and reason'. If we look up, we see this famous quote being written, erased, and reinscribed in chalk on the ceiling by a ghostly holographic hand. On the floor beneath, a ghostly left foot writes Henri Bergson's words: 'Many diverse images, borrowed from very different orders of things, may, by the convergence of their action, direct the consciousness to the precise point where there is a certain intuition to be seized.'

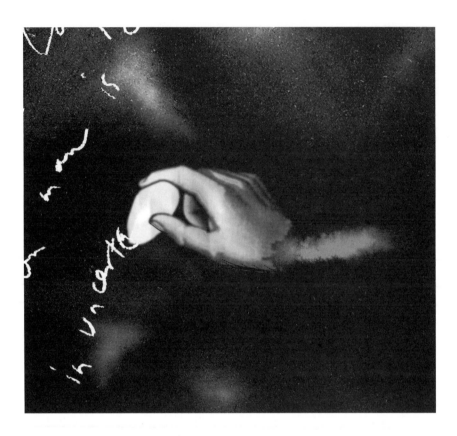

What intuition is to be seized from the diverse images here in the first room, the constellation which converges on the theme of immersion? A black and white photograph of an adult male steeped and stupefied in a bath of milk is connected to the exhibits around it by vectors.

To the left, a group of grim engravings depicting dudhputti, the Indian practice (long since banned, I'm happy to say) of drowning baby girls in milk. To the right, several buoyant images and reports of Cleopatra, Beau Brummel and others who sought to rejuvenate themselves by bathing in milk. Laser beams connect the wall-mounted displays to a free-standing animatronic head of Jane Ellen Harrison reading from her ground-

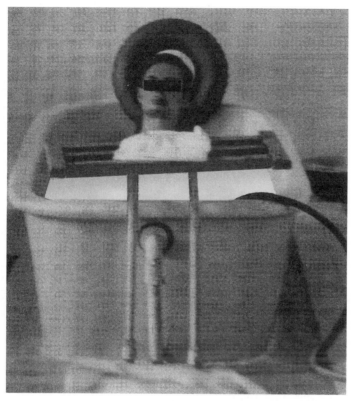

breaking study of ancient mystery rites, *Prolegomena to the Study of Greek Religion* (1903): 'The question remains – what was the exact ritual of the falling into milk? ... Did the neophyte actually fall into a bath of milk... ?' Her voice has a compelling urgency to it which makes us consider the question without any irritable reaching after an answer. Instead of a caption, a hand-typed manuscript from Wellcome's collection, entitled 'Some Notes on the History of Milk' by A. W. Harris, stands beside her under a bell jar on a plinth, open to the page shown overleaf.

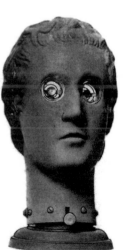

old milking songs of Scotland.

(Note. I think perhaps we could get some
of these songs. A.W.H.)

At her birth St. Bridget was bathed in milk, and this
takes us once more back to ancient pagan religious rites.
In the primitive baptismal rites of Ancient Greece not only
was there a ritual act of drinking milk, but evidence
strongly suggests that in those days the neophyte was also
immersed in a bath of milk. For this there is a useful
parallel from Egyptian ritual, and the survival is
indicated by St. Bridget's similar experience.

That bathing in milk was also a death rite is shown
both in traditional ballad lore, and in traditional games.
In the beautiful ballad of Burd Ellen is the verse :-

"Tak up, tak up my bonny young son,
Gar wash him wi' the milk.
Tak up, tak up my fair lady,
Gar row her in the silk."

So too, in the children's game of Green Gravel, where
the general movements of the game show that it is derived from
an ancient funeral rite, the most constant formulae in the
game-rhymes include the line -

"Wash them in milk, and clothe them in silk."

Men of the mediaeval period, as indeed of almost every

As we read, recordings of children playing the game Green Gravel, and of minstrels singing 'Burd Ellen', mingle strangely with Harrison's voice, making the hair on the backs of our necks rise. Another vector links the foregoing items to a trench in the floor filled with what is in fact latex emulsion. (For obvious reasons milk would not be practical, as it would 'turn', requiring constant replacement. However, the smell of rotting cheese is wafted into the space from concealed vents. The evocative potency of olfactory data will be utilised throughout the exhibition.) The white paint in the trench serves as a screen on to which *Nosferatu*, the film by F. W. Murnau, made in 1922 and starring the incomparable Max Schreck as the eponymous vampire (a.k.a. Count Dracula), is projected from a source directly overhead. (A note informs us that 'Nosferatu' means 'splashed with milk' in Transylvanian – the link between vampirism and nursing will be explored in greater depth anon.)

The dudhputti engravings are linked to an oleograph from Wellcome's collection of the holy cow personified as World Mother with many Sanskrit verses (and one phrase in English). Progressive enlargements focus on a figure inside the cow's transparent udder, waist-deep in milk (overleaf).

Already I think we can appreciate how the constellation method works.

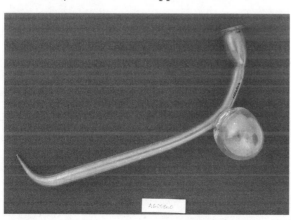

The intuition we seize is that milk is a matter of life and death. Our beginnings are in it, but also more than a whiff of our end. An immersion in milk is an initiation. For many of us, one birth is not enough.

Miniature Breast Pump for pets (shown twice actual size)

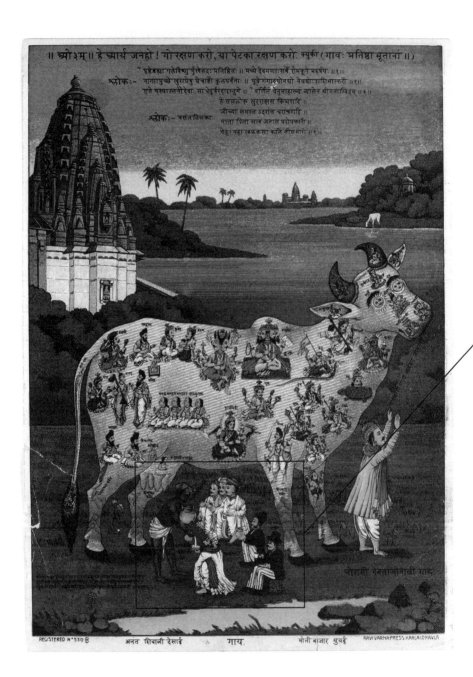

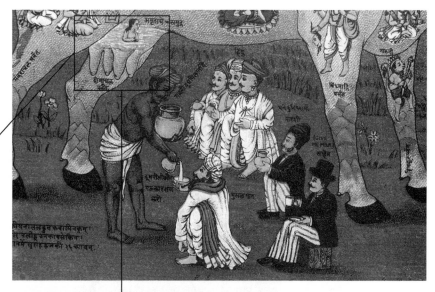

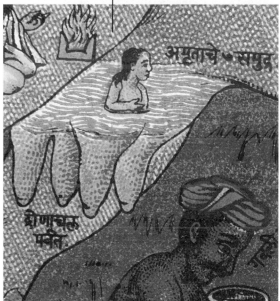

↑
Detail, enlarged, from the oleograph showing a farmer giving milk to Hindus, Parsees and Englishmen. One of the latter says "GIVE ME MILK".

←
Detail, further enlarged, showing someone deeply into milk.

THE SECOND ROOM

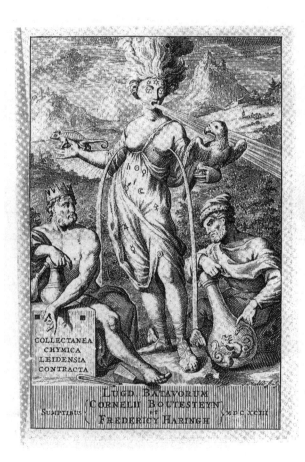

A notice above the door warns us that we may find some of the exhibits behind the heavy velvet drapes disturbing. The split-screen projection on show within is a collage of what are normally considered incompatible genres, a visual cacophony. It's shocking to see matters of the deepest gravity clash with trivia, hype, pornography, kitsch and comedy as they do here. Medical footage of breast surgery, radical and cosmetic, is juxtaposed with a clip of Barbara Windsor losing her bikini top, with Jayne Mansfield cradling a pair of milk bottles, with images of polybreasted goddesses and supernumerary mammae, with a peep through a keyhole at an anonymous prostitute pleasuring a client *à l'espagnol*, with advertisements for bras and bondage gear, with footage of prosthetic breasts or with the scene from Woody Allen's *Everything You Always Wanted to Know About Sex But Were Afraid to Ask* (1972) in which the nerdy little comic is pursued by a gigantic spurting mammary gland. Examples of postmastectomy nudes photographed mostly by women – some celebrating strength and defiance, others mourning loss – are at one end of an emotional spectrum, at the other end of which breasts are eroticised and exploited, mostly by men. In *Un Chien Andalou*[3] a man in a trance of agony/ecstasy kneads an unenthusiastic woman's breasts, which suddenly become her buttocks. Elsewhere in the montage a man morphs into 'The Breast', enacting the unlikely premise of a novella by Philip Roth: 'Just as they are able to increase the milk yield of cows with injections of the lactogenic agent gH, the growth hormone, so it has been hypothesized that I could very possibly become a milk-producing mammary gland with the appropriate stimulation.' (Philip Roth, *The Breast*)

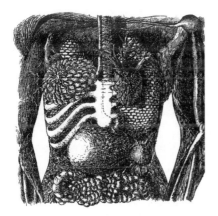 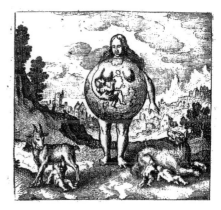

3 Salvador Dali and Luis Buñuel (1928)

Breast-envy and breast-fear in males may be traceable to unconscious
memories of the less differentiated state we all knew as infants. Here's
Samuel Ferris MD, writing about breasts in 1783:

> Notwithstanding the secretion of milk, for the purposes of nature, is
> confined to the female of every species of the whole class: yet men
> possess glands of a similar structure, and which are capable, in some
> degree, of a similar office. A ferous and turbid liquor, like milk, may be
> drawn from the breasts of almost all new born infants, male and female.
> Neither is the capability of affording such a liquor, at all times quickly
> lost. It has been drawn from the breasts of children of both sexes at
> different ages, five months, two years, nine years old and upward.
> – Samuel Ferris MD, *A Dissertation on Milk*, Edinburgh, 1783

This transgressive theme is pursued in exhibits among which are several
examples of males developing breasts and lactating, due to sympathy[4],
exigency[5] or hormonal imbalance[6]. The significance in this context of a clip

---

4 'What else can I say about my parents? Even though Mama was vigorous and authoritarian, she couldn't breastfeed
us, because the doctor had put her on a homeogalactotherapeutic cure in which she drank part of her own milk while
forming the rest into small cheeses which she smeared over her body in order to maintain the softness of her skin.
What father was ever more dedicated to his family? With a prodigious will, Papa managed to give milk, and not a skim
milk poor in nutritional value but a thick and creamy milk. And thus the three of us... were breastfed by Papa until we
were old enough to marry, my two older sisters hanging from the two regulation breasts and I, the smallest, hanging
from an extra breast he had grown for the occasion on his shoulder and which our family doctor wanted to cut off,
maintaining that it was a lipoma. Feeding times coincided with office hours, and in the ministry he set a good example
for all, a zealous employee who with one hand carried out his duties while with the other he gave suck to his daughters.'
Alberto Savinio, *The Lives of the Gods*, trans. James Brook, Atlas, 1991

5 Coleridge, in his *Notebooks*, writes about a book he has been reading, Sir John Franklin's *The Narrative of a Journey to the
Shores of the Polar Sea, in the Years 1819, 20, 21, and 22*: 'The story of the Indian husband suckling his infant, tells (157-8) of
a "young Chipewyan"who "descended to the office of nurse, so degrading in the eyes of a Chipewyan, as partaking of the
duties of a woman", and "by the force of the powerful passion" with which he tended his son, "a flow of milk actually took
place from his breast..."'
The Notebooks of S. T. Coleridge, ed. by Kathleen Coburn and Merton Christensen, Vol. 4, 1819–1826, NOTES

6 Cf. *Man Made, A Memoir of My Body*, by Ken Baker. Baker's memoir about struggling with masculinity in contemporary
culture is unique. Throughout his adolescence and early adult life, he suffered from a massive overabundance of prolactin –
the hormone that allows females to produce milk. This imbalance, caused by a benign tumor in Baker's brain, engendered a
host of physical problems, such as impotence, excess fat on his hips and breasts and sensitive nipples that would
occasionally excrete a milky substance.' Agent, Jane Dystel. Copyright 2001 Cahners Business Information, Inc.

from Tod Browning's *Dracula*, 1931, in which Bela Lugosi transforms himself into a bat, is less puzzling when we're told that the male Dyak fruit bat not only lactates but suckles its young. (A note informs us that the link between vampirism and nursing will be explored further anon.)

Tearing ourselves away from these we enter a placid vestibule in which images of women breast-feeding babies are displayed. Yes, we think, seeing treatments of this primal theme by artists from various times and places reveals cultural differences while emphasising our common humanity. Edifying.

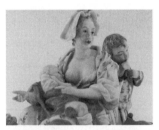

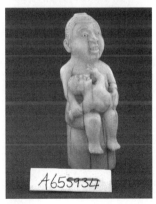

White negroes Black caucasians

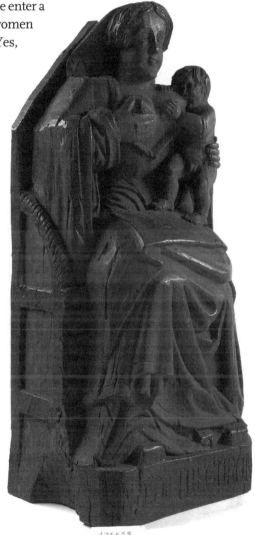

But, hark! This little male babe pipes a
subversive ditty from a speaker hidden
in his head. We bend closer to hear:

From north to south, from east to west,
for feeding babies, breast is best.
As an infant, I agree
mother's breast is best for me.
But her submission to my bent
provides me more than nourishment.
Baby whales and baby bats
drink in minerals and fats,
but I absorb a paradigm
which will haunt me for all time.
Milk is why we're given lips
and why we form relationships.
What is kissing, after all,
but nursing that is mutual?

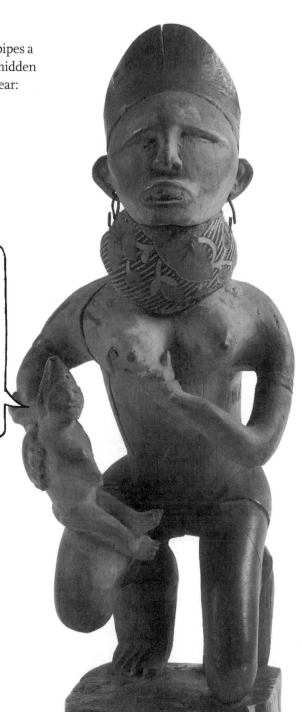

THE THIRD ROOM

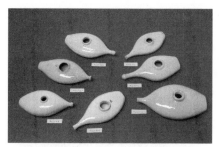

Wellcome's collection includes a variety of feeding bottles, surrogates for the breast. How elegant and modern this porcelain flotilla looks compared to this fanciful bird-bottle. They must all have felt cold, hard and ungiving enough in the mouths of the recently weaned to establish the foundation for future breast-nostalgias. Don't you think?

Wellcome's collection also includes a variety of surrogates for the living nipple. Before rubber existed, capping a baby's feeding

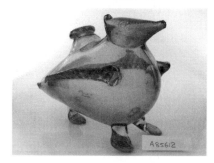

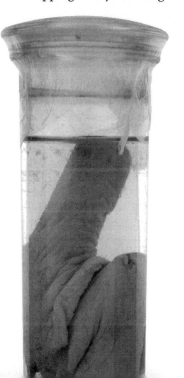

bottle with a teat of real veal, cut from a calf's udder, would have made no one shudder. We can see past our initial distaste and appreciate the resourcefulness of pre-industrial homesteaders who hit on this expedient when we consider the tough-love alternative of the feeding horn which, while having an associative connection

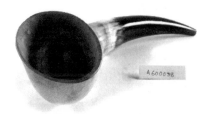

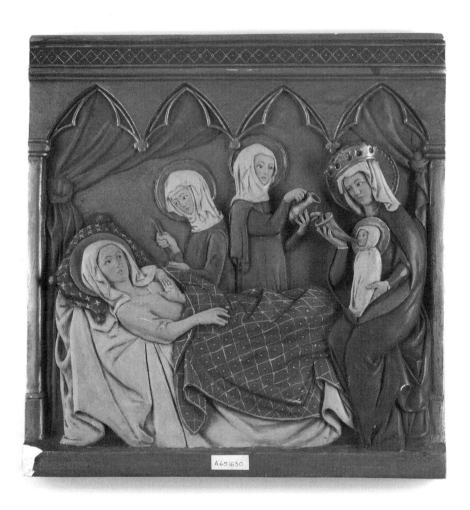

A651630

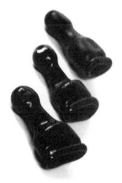

with the cow, must have seemed a brutal intrusion into the toothless mouths of infants accustomed to the warmth and softness of the maternal breast.

The historical teats on display include this vulcanised trio. A traditional method of weaning among light-skinned peoples was to blacken the breast, a form of aversion therapy. (It seems logical to suppose that a black mother might whiten her breast and put her child off just as effectively, though the fact that milk itself is white might complicate matters.) Babies accustomed to suckling at a white breast probably found weaning more of a wrench when the surrogate teat was black, but there was no help for white folks back in the days when these teats were made. Like Model T Fords, rubber back then was available in any colour as long as it was

black. Years later, teats like the JOLLY GRIP-TIGHT FAMILY, riding high on their crescent-shaped biberon, were cast in transluscent amber rubber, racially ambiguous, strong enough to withstand repeated sterilisation.

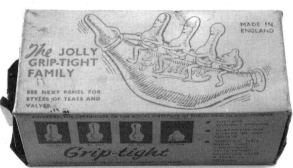

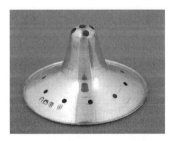

The caption implies that this is a prosthetic nipple forged in gold, but we know better. It reads: 'A serpent fastens itself to Caradog Freichfra, and can only be allured away by his wife Tegau offering it one of her breasts, "of which she loses the nipple when the beast is cut off. The defect being replaced with gold, she is ever after known as Tegau Eur-fron, Tegau of the golden breast".' (John Rhys, *Celtic Folklore*, Welsh and Many, Oxford, 1901)

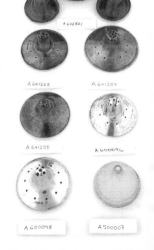

But we weren't born yesterday. We know a nipple shield when we see one. Or when we see many. Beautiful, aren't they?

Nipples are incredible.
Babies think they're edible.
Tender after being chewed,
after being drained of food,
the throbbing buds cannot abide
abrasion, so they have to hide,
withdrawn, if only for a spell,
like a whelk into its shell.
The nipple sleeps, its eyes are sealed,
protected by a nipple-shield.

You're getting tired, I can see you're starting to flag. Anticipating this, we've set up a Milk Bar at precisely this point, where refreshing dairy products – yogurts, cheeses, curds and whey, plus a whole spectrum of milks, from the blue of skimmed to the gold of buttermilk – can be sampled. The milk-wine known as koumiss, a staple on the Russian steppes for centuries, will restore the spring to your step.

THE MILK BAR

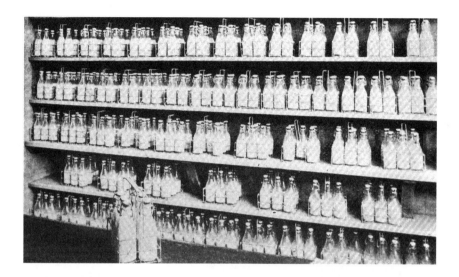

	Human	Cow	Porpoise	Mare	Hamoose	Goat	Ass	Ewe	Sow
Specific Gravity	·	·	about 1000.0	1034.9	1035.4	1032.9			
Fat . . .	3.5	3.9	45.80	1.09	5.56	4.3	1.6	6.8	4.8
Sugar . .	6.5	4.7	1.33	6.65	5.41	4.0	6.1	4.8	3.4
Proteids . .	1.6	3.7	11.19	1.89	3.86	4.6	2.2	6.3	1.3
Ash . . .	0.25	0.7	0.57	0.31	1.03	0.6	0.5	0.8	0.9
Tot'l Solids	11.80	13.0	58.89	9.94	15.86	13.5	10.4	18.7	15.4
Analyst			F. Purdie	Vieth	Richmond & Payne				

And look, here's a menu of milks of many mammals you can try, showing their relative constituents. Tired? Yes, one does get tired. Of milk. Of oneself. Experts agree. After all this research, passive and active, the dangers are '... fatigue, introspection, disillusionment, eclipse of an overview, corrosion of confidence, and mixed emotions attendant upon any long and troubled intimacy.'[7]

7 Judith Thurman, 'Siren Songs', *New Yorker*, 3 September 2001

THE FOURTH ROOM

"Every value evokes its opposite and is in constant struggle with it."
– Gaston Bachelard

That's the quote above the door to the next room. I painted all the quotes myself, by hand. Some nights, after everyone has gone, I wander through the empty exhibition in the company of my spiritual mentors, Walter Benjamin and Gaston Bachelard. I take a brush and a pot of enamel and go around retouching the quotes the public has smudged, or in some

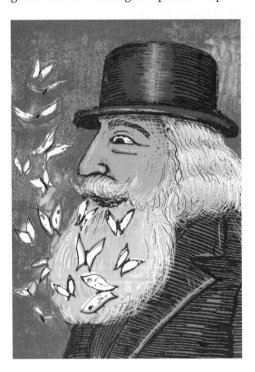

cases defaced. Tonight Bachelard points out that quote of his above the door. It's been smudged. When I'm done he nods approval. He reminds me of Walt Whitman. His grey beard full of butterflies... Bachelard! I salute you!

Great phenomenologist of the material imagination, you who psychoanalysed the four elements and prophesised that someone someday would write a 'psychoanalysis of beverages' which 'must present the dialectic of alcohol and milk, of milk and water, of Dionysus against Cybele'.[8]

---

8 Gaston Bachelard, *Water and Dreams, An Essay on the Imagination of Matter*, trans. Edith R. Farrell, Dallas, 1983

You didn't mean that I would write it, did you, Gaston? You shake your grey head, no. Thank God for that! After this, I hope to be done with milk forever. Our laughter echoes in the empty room. Not empty. The room is full of snakes. Images of snakes, and the sound of them hatching and hissing. Look, here's the serpent tempting Adam and Eve. Look, it has the face of a child and the withered dugs of a crone.

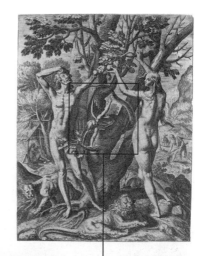

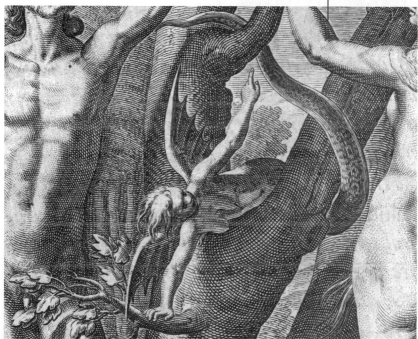

And over here's an image taken from the bookplate of The Sanitary Institute pasted on the inside front cover of *Analysis of Milk and Milk Products*, by Leffmann and Beam, 1896, in the Wellcome Library.

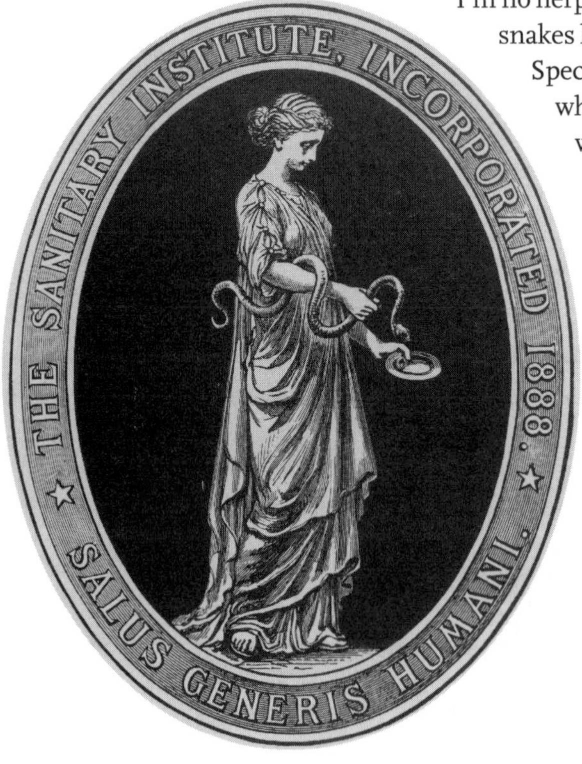

I'm no herpatologist, but I've heard that snakes love milk. I've read 'The Speckled Band', for instance, in which a saucer of milk is a clue which helps Sherlock Holmes identify the murder weapon: an adder. We'll come back to Holmes in a minute. But first, let's consider the image of someone filling his/her mouth with milk in order to squirt it through a bamboo tube down the gullet of a snake. This seems to have been the purpose of the object shown here.

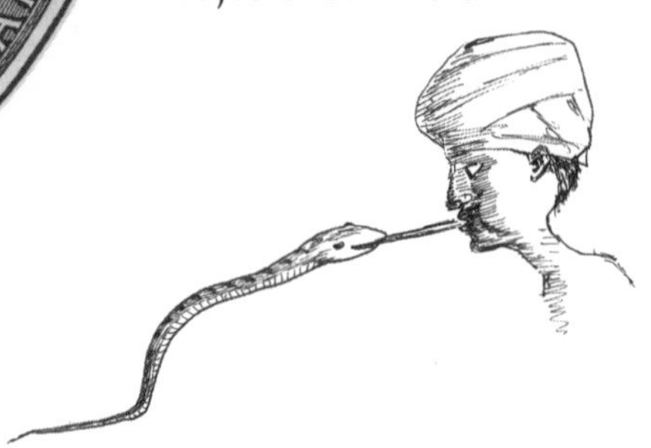

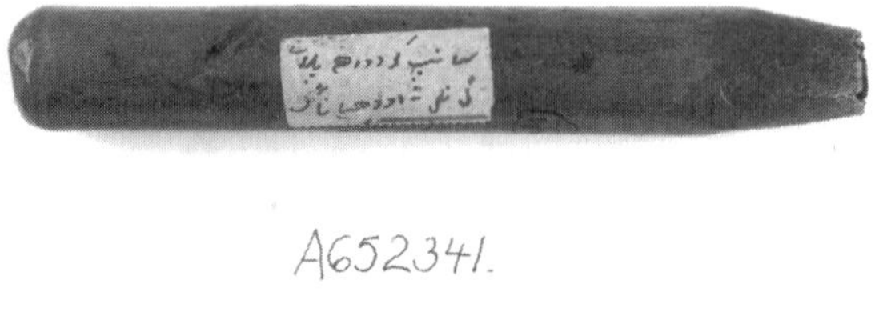

'Probably from the Middle East, probably second half of the nineteenth century.' The idea appeals to the imagination as a reversal of the natural order, an inversion of the tired cliché of a snake injecting someone with venom. Inversions are one of the simplest forms of imagination and one of the most powerful. 'In order to see the things of this world correctly, you have got to look at them all upside down.' (Balthesar Gracian, 1601–56) 'Without contraries is no progression.' (William Blake)

In the Milk Exhibition's constellation of reversals we find:

- lactation of males
- animals suckling humans
- humans suckling animals
- adults being breast-fed.

But let's return now, as promised, to Sherlock Holmes, and to the vampire theme. To a more fundamental reversal of the natural order of things:

While they were talking a sudden cry of pain was heard, Nurse and master rushed together to the nursery. Imagine his feelings, Mr. Holmes, as he saw his wife rise from a kneeling position beside the cot and saw blood upon the child's exposed neck and upon the sheet. With a cry of horror, he turned his wife's face to the light and saw blood all round her lips. It was she – beyond all question – who had drunk the poor baby's blood.
– Arthur Conan Doyle, 'The Case of the Sussex Vampire'

Don't worry. It turns out that the mother is sucking the poison out of a wound inflicted by a toxic dart. She's vindicated. But the point is that the image of a mother sucking the lifeblood from her child refreshes our interest in milk. It satisfies our thirst for revenge. How dare things resist us so stubbornly? (Walter Benjamin reminds me to tell you that the German word for object, *gegenstand*, literally means counter-stand, resistance.)

How dare milk be so white?

The pure whiteness of milk was a matter of considerable wonder to all peoples, and is repeatedly alluded to in the folklore and riddles of the world.

– Benjamin Walker, *Encyclopedia of Esoteric Man*

Bachelard:

It is not absurd to speak of the blackness of milk, if one feels that white becomes white by repulsing darkness.

Another voice interjects:

Although milk seems to be white in color, due to the reflection and dispersion of light in the fat globules and other solids, actually it is faintly yellow... Certain American paper money is printed in yellow because of this basic hue of milk...

– S. J. Crumbine and J. A. Tobey, *The Most Nearly Perfect Food* (*The Story of Milk*)

Uno Holmberg can't resist informing us of the three Luonnotars, deities in Finnish mythology who appear

... in the songs on the origin of iron, in which it is described how their milk was allowed by them to run into the earth, one dripping forth black milk, the second white, the third blood-red; the first giving birth to smithy-iron, the second to steel, and the third to refuse iron.

– Uno Holmberg, *Mythology of All Races*

And then, Paul Celan, his voice tolling like a knell in the rafters:

Black milk of daybreak we drink it at nightfall / we drink it at noon in the morning we drink it at night / drink it and drink it

– Paul Celan, 'Death Fugue'

Silence! Will you please be quiet! These voices in my head, of course, imagined. The Milk Exhibition, imaginary, a constellation of synapses, a collage of images projected on to an interior screen, a fantasy spun out to compensate, to console me for my failure, for the paucity of...

I seek revenge. By exposing the corruption at the core of that which is traditionally most white, most pure, most 'innocent': milk. The image of black milk insults reason, it resonates as more than a mere topsy-turvy conceit, it's a horror, an obscenity commensurate with the obscenity of the truth, my failure, our species' betrayal of its potential. Our collective failure to evolve, to cut the cord, to move on, to mature.

Look on these works, ye mighty, and despair!

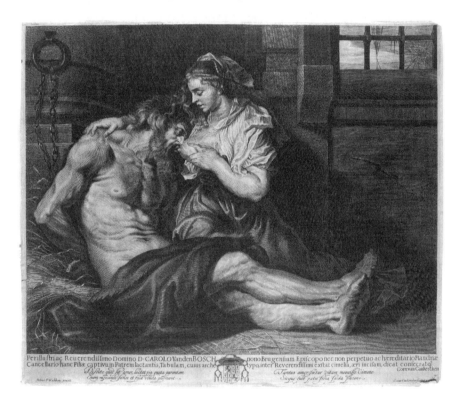

Images of adults, male and female, still at it! Still nursing at the breast! Uninitiated, unweaned! There's hope, as Kafka said, but not for us.

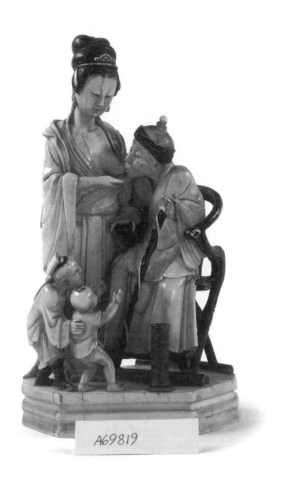

A69819

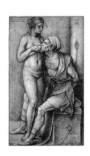

My old man makes a last request:
to be fed like a baby at his mama's breast.
I take him to a fancy restaurant,
I say "Daddy, you can order anything you want."
Unless a man has a loss to mourn
he hasn't been born at all.
Until a woman's been intimate with grief
she's still a little girl.

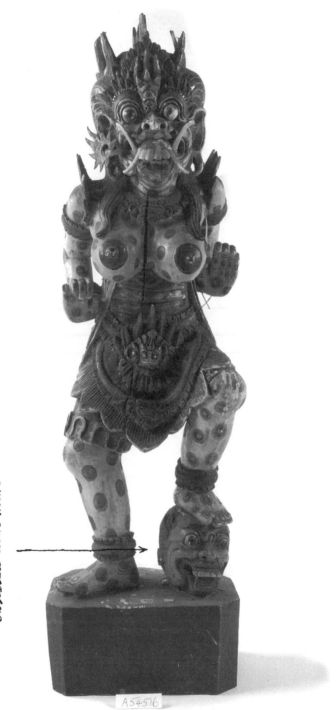

Obsessed with milk.

A54516

I want to say 'it's finished'.

I want to say I'm done with milk. To get past it, as if it were an obstacle in my path. It is. Milk is in my way. I came across it in the course of my development which was arrested at the point where I fell into it. How to extricate myself? Immersed in it, drunk on it, I experience the 'white out' which Arctic explorers report when blinded in blizzards, disorientated by a sky and ground of uniform opaque whiteness without end, without horizon, without depth...

In despair, I drink my ink and write the rest in milk...

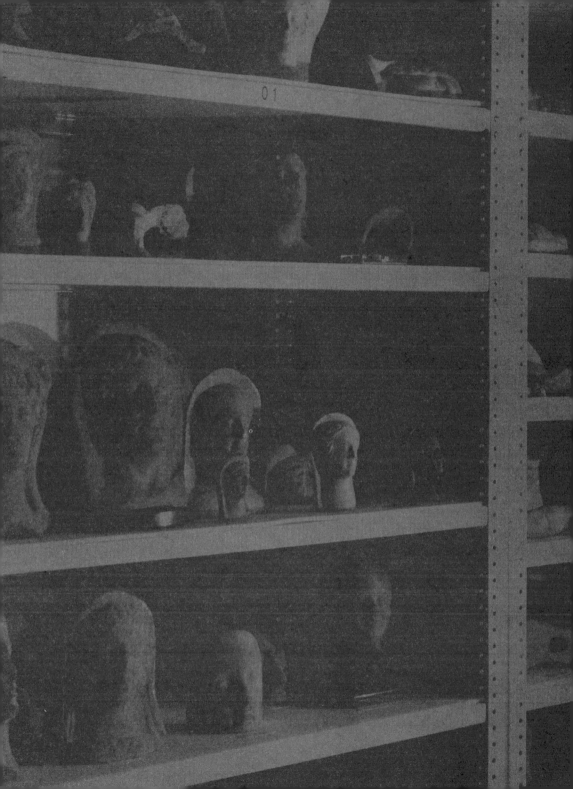

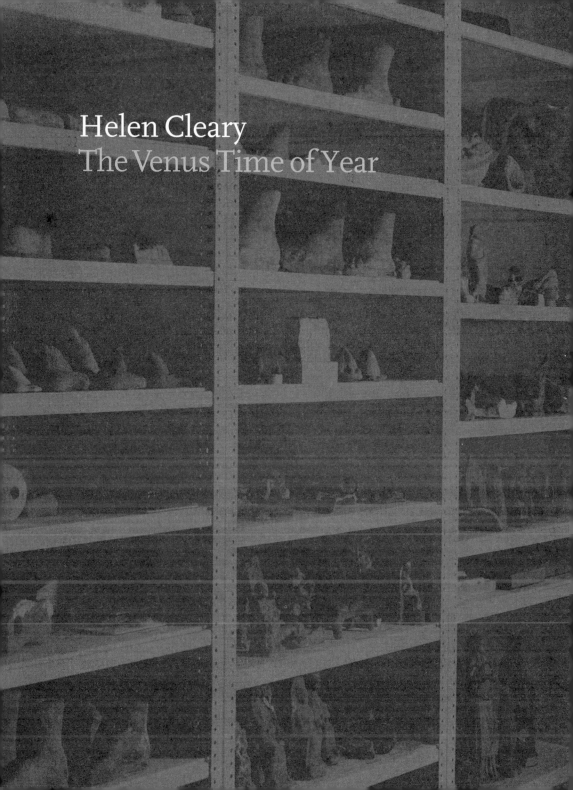

Helen Cleary
The Venus Time of Year

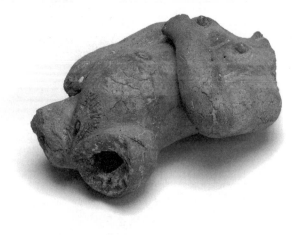

S UZY IS ALONE IN THE TOP-STOREY FLAT with the windows wide open to city sounds, the intermittent wail of sirens and the trundle and screech of trains along the three lines that corner the block. The Big Smoke is airless; it's humid and the kitchen in particular is oily with heat. She's preparing a meal, that ancient industry. Anchovies preserved in sunflower oil. Mushrooms cooked first in butter. Crème fraîche. Fresh tarragon, but in moderation. She takes a single leaf between her lips so she can savour the surprisingly modern tang of aniseed. Which reminds her of the school exchange trip to Normandy. Clandestine slurps of pastis turned milky with water. Where did they buy it, her and Kirsty? They were fourteen; no one would have sold them alcohol surely? Whatever. Their kisses were so delicious it was worth the risk. (*Oh Kirsty, why did I let you get away?*) She sips from her long-stemmed glass, legal now. She has to have wine while she prepares a meal; it's a habit that lends sophistication. *When we are grown-ups...* She's young enough still to relish the advantages bestowed by adulthood.

She opens a cupboard door, kneels down to find the big orange-red pot – a Le Creuset inherited from her mother – and sets it over the blue gas flame, then fills it with boiling water from the kettle. Steam tumbles over the lip of the pot and mists the splashback. In go bunches of fresh tagliatelle, soft and papery like powdered skin, and the bubbling water is momentarily checked as the pasta warms.

The front door bangs shut. Running footsteps.

'Hi! Suzy!'

'Hey, Barney! You're home late.' She turns to greet him.

'Mum got stuck at work! I went to DJ's.' He flings his school bag on the floor and wipes beads of perspiration from his upper lip.

And there she is, Cal, Barney's mum, standing behind him, hands on his shoulders for a second before he squirms out of reach. 'Sorry we're late, Suz,' she says, all big eyes and mischief at the corners of her mouth. This vision of Cal affects Suzy's stomach with a lurch and a plunge – still, after three years of living together. Suzy abandons her cooking and goes to her girlfriend, takes a handful of the other woman's T-shirt at the waist, and pulls her in to plant a kiss on her cheek and neck, beneath the jaw. Cal laughs and returns affection. They embrace, Cal's breasts just below Suzy's own.

'Aw! Yuk-a-yuk. You two!' Barney turns from the sink where he is filling a glass with water. He screws up his face. This isn't awkward or heartfelt; it's any kid's response to such an amorous exchange and so public. He's seen it all before, but he never fails to register distaste, not these days.

'Sorry Barnabas. You can have a cuddle too if you want.' Cal leers at him, crossing her eyes and pouting her lips.

'No way, Mum. Time's up. I got business to attend to.' And he gulps down the entire glass of water in one go and runs from the kitchen. Suzy and Cal look at each other. He'll be on his computer again. There's nothing they can do to lure him away. They've tried everything. They don't even bother to discuss it any more.

'Will he eat anchovies d'you think?'

'Sure. He'll eat anything as long as you don't ask him beforehand. Never give him the choice.'

'You're a hard woman.' Suzy returns to her work, chopping the anchovies small, hoping they'll get lost in the pasta. Anything visibly alien and Barney might pick out the pieces, piling tiny corpses on the side of his plate. She stirs the tagliatelle. Only a couple more minutes and it'll be done. This is a simple meal, easy to make, but surprisingly rich. Something special for a Friday night.

'Shall we give the boys a call?'

'Yeah. Why not. You do it. I'll finish this.'

Cal goes into the hall, picks up the receiver and dials. Dan and Leo live three storeys down and the two couples often spend a Friday or Saturday night together, eating, playing cards and drinking into the small hours. Barney likes having them around and Cal thinks it's good for him. As he gets older she worries about role models, even though he sees his father once a week, minimum. Suzy tells her he's doing fine, but she can see that Cal has a point. From the hall comes Cal's murmured phone conversation and laughter. 'They'll be up in a sec,' she says as she enters the kitchen again. She sits on a high stool, the only chair that fits the space, and stretches her arms over her head.

'My back's killing me.'

'I'll get the massage oil out later.'

'Is that a threat or a promise?' And they pull a face at each other.

Cal shifts her bum on the stool, trying to get comfortable. 'I had a terrible day.'

'What happened?'

'A breech birth. The father panicked. He practically strangled one of the nurses.'

'Typical.'

'Well. First child and everything.'

'But you sorted him out?'

'Yeah. I sorted them all out.'

'No court case this week then.'

Cal sighs. 'Not this week.'

Suzy places a colander in the sink and lifts the heavy pan from the hob, pouring away the water expertly, her wrist protected from the hot steam by a tea-towel. Ribbons of pasta slip from the pan and coil in the colander. She turns back to the hob and finishes off her sauce.

'How was your day anyway, Suzy Sue?'

'Oh, you know. Fair to middling. I got some words down at least.' Suzy always feels guilty when Cal asks. Cal works so hard, such long hours at the hospital, with a hellish commute either end of her shift. Suzy, on the other hand, gets up, has a leisurely breakfast, a shower if she feels like it, and then, when she's ready, switches on her computer and bashes away at the keyboard. *Hopefully.* She won't admit as much, but she's barely been able to concentrate of late. She's managed thirty thousand words and she's run out of steam; she's reached a cerebral cul-de-sac. Bad news, especially as she had only just sorted herself out after the previous year (which had been hell) and got back on course to complete. Now her funding has all but disappeared and things are getting desperate. She should take a part-time job, but she's scared she'll abandon her PhD altogether if she does that.

Even though she's planned meticulously, chapter by chapter, her mind keeps wandering. She's intrigued by a recent find – one of the terracotta figurines, a female nude. It's not the best of thousands she's set eyes on over the last four years, but it's such an expressive piece. Headless, missing an arm and both legs from mid-thigh down, she's still beautiful, this nude: the curve of pregnant belly and protruding navel as emphatic as a full stop; the pronounced vulva, clitoris on display (an exclamation mark), pubic hair painstakingly represented; swollen breasts, caressed by the left hand; and a muscled arm. Very human. Very tender. This is a celebration of fecundity. All woman; a woman in love with her own body. And she's set Suzy thinking. Who made her? No man surely, and no entrepreneur; it's not one of the mass-produced votive body parts and mother figures, some of them made in moulds and probably sold by the dozen outside temples and shrines. This one would have been offered to Diana or Venus or one of the *matronae*, left with a prayer or a plea-bargain. *Give me a good birth and I'll worship you forever.* Suzy's theory is she's a one-off, fashioned by hand, not in a mould, and lovingly so. She's British too and there aren't many examples from Roman Britain.

*

Slowly night descended following dusk, that goddess in her frail silk robes the colour of birds' new feathers. This was when Aelia would walk alone, walking hard, hoping to shrug lust off. Yes, it was *that* time of year again.

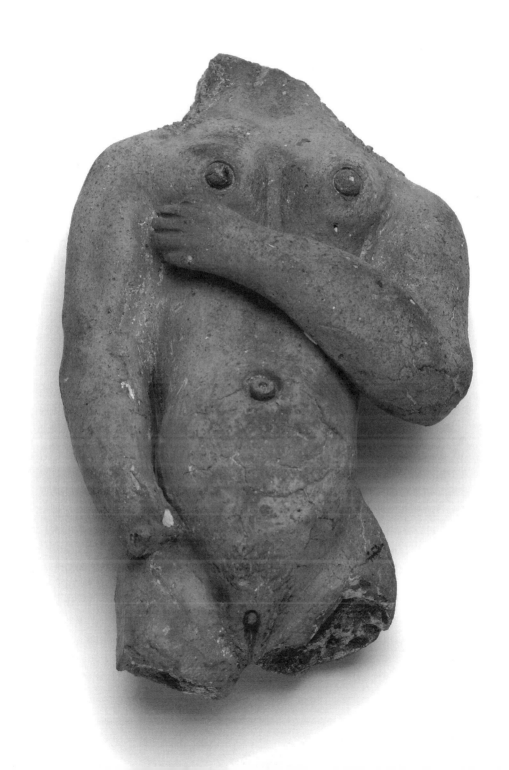

Always in the summer. The last two summers at least. Why? Because of the vanilla stink of gorse blossom warmed by long hours of sun. Airborne, the flowers' scent crept through the night and, this, the smell of lust (Venus's perfume), became trapped in her blanket, malingering there, persistent as a disease. Aelia slept badly, her waking dreams vivid with body parts: men and women, naked and tangled together in Bacchanalian ecstasy; grasping hands, taut legs, the sway of balls, belly and breast. Sometimes it was dawn before she finally lost consciousness, only to wake a few hours later, exhausted.

So before she went to bed she would walk. Nobody stopped her. She stepped between the houses and wooden outbuildings, along the pathway carved through the copse, and past the dewpond, where she collected watercress and moss growing in fringes along the cool banks. She came to open fenland and took the drove road they'd built, the long straight road which led to the town and ended at the foot of the municipal tower. At first people had been scared of this big wide road. No one had ever seen anything like it, so perfect, unwavering. They wondered if the spirits might use it as a route back to the world of the living. That was years ago – before she was born, before her father even came to this island. She was not afraid. She walked and watched her shadow walking too, the wide sky up above like a band of quartz.

But it was no good. Both darkness and light caressed her limbs. She admired herself, sucked at her own flesh, licked her shoulder, the pellet of bone there where the arm began. She mumbled at the sinew on her inside wrist, leaving behind a trail of saliva, a sliver of kiss. *Taste the life-salt. What might a man taste of? Let me know, O Venus. Let me discover him soon. Lead me there.* Oh how she wanted. She wanted so much she caved in. She'd get down on the ground, foetal with want, the wet grasses and clover by her face. And she'd hold onto herself. There, in that place. Later, in the twilight, she would walk back, grass-seeds stuck to her cheeks. She'd sneak into their living quarters, tiptoeing past her father asleep in his chair, and undress, fumbling in the dark.

And the days? Just as agonising. She might stop working and look about her and she was consumed again. Dappled light between leaf and branch suggested passion. Silver and iron threaded through the stream became a twist of swimming lovers. Summer's heat congealed in the air, and with summer's heat came the delicious prickle of sweat down back and inside thighs. The sky – blue, blue sky – was as intense as her longing. Even when she was with her father, helping him as he dug clay from the marl pit or prepared a fire for the kiln (and this had to be done with care), she might be seized with desire. She had no words for what she felt, only images. But she didn't want her father to know. It wasn't that she was ashamed; she just didn't want to admit that one day she might leave him and start a new life, a married life. Perhaps if there had been a woman with them things might have been different, but her mother had died shortly after childbirth, rotting from the inside. As a baby, she'd been raised on goat's milk. No one had expected her to survive more than a few weeks, let alone fifteen years.

*

Before Suzy and Cal can get to the door, Barney has run from his room to welcome the visitors.

'High five!'

Barney hesitates. 'That's so out. Look, you do this.' And he takes Dan's hand and directs him in a complex series of gestures, linking thumbs and brushing knuckles.

'I knew that.' Dan grins and hastily withdraws his hand, unable to follow the boy. 'How's it hanging, anyway, tiger?'

'All right. Guess what? I've got to the bit where they're on the helicopter and the water explodes with bombs and stuff. Come and have a go.' Dan looks at the two women in the kitchen doorway. He's sheepish. He loves Barney's computer games almost as much as Barney does, and he's dying to play, but he knows better – Barney shouldn't be encouraged, not without permission at least.

Cal rolls her eyes. 'Okay. Two minutes, that's your lot. I'll lay the table and then' – she considers her threat – '... then you've got to come and make conversation with us. Just imagine.' But they're not listening. Dan is jostling Barney to be first through the bedroom door.

'Bless,' says Leo as he approaches and kisses Cal then Suzy on both cheeks. He hands them a bottle of wine. 'This should keep us going.'

'Cheers.' And Suzy puts it to one side. 'Glass of Chardonnay first?'

He nods. 'So, you two horny love-muffins, it's the weekend! Thank the lord above.'

'I know. It's been a pig of week.'

'Tell me about it. I'm ready to throw in the towel.'

'You think you've got it hard. I do life or death, honey. Several times a day.' Cal tickles him and he bearhugs her so that her feet leave the floor. Her slender frame looks childlike against his big, gym-toned body. Cal shrieks and tries to punch his back. And Suzy watches them from her side of the small room. They seem miles away, on another planet. She gets a rush of jealousy, as if she'd knocked an old bruise. Cal hasn't always gone for women; she was *married* for Christ's sake.

*

Her kneeling father used birch tongues to dip an unglazed pot in a vat of slip. His head was bowed and the muscles in his forearms flexed then relaxed with the effort of controlled movement. It was so hot he'd left off his long vest. They were not formal together, not when they were working. She went up behind him, put her hands over his eyes and kissed him on the crown. He laughed and put down the dripping pot with precision, not needing to see, then he peeled away her fingers, one by one.

She offered to bring him drinking water. How could she have anticipated his thirst? Aelia, my faithful daughter, he said and smiled at her, crow's-feet settling around his eyes and mouth. He had begun to age or she had begun to notice the details: silver hair at his temples, the skin lined and red at his neck. But his body remained strong. She didn't have to worry yet.

She stepped from the workshop into bright sunshine before entering the shade of the kitchen. She went to the storeroom, ladled water into a drinking cup and returned to his side. They continued to work and eventually she asked if they would be ready for market. He replied that it depended on her output. He was teasing, but he'd been watching her closely of late. He must have been aware that her mind was wandering – maybe he knew where it was wandering to – but he hadn't said anything.

She hesitated, then asked the question she had wanted to ask for months. She wanted to go with him. Was it possible? A shadow passed across his face. He wasn't sure. It was such a distance and – but he floundered to find more reasons why not. She begged him. She had never seen the town. Eventually he conceded that he would consider her proposal. Perhaps they would find accommodation, so she could rest and return the next day.

Almost as good as a promise. Now she was flushed with excitement. She might go to the town, and if she went to the town she could visit the temple, say her prayers and submit a token to Venus. If her prayers were heard she might find love – it was possible that her lover was there, waiting for her to arrive, although he didn't know it. There were men in the village, boys her own age that her father had introduced her to, but she had turned away, indignant. She knew them so well, too well. They wouldn't do. Her father hadn't pursued the matter. Aelia suspected he was afraid of pushing her away. He didn't want to lose her altogether. How could he have so much as contemplated one of them as her husband? They were not potters; they were smallholders, keeping sheep or working arable plots. Their wives and sisters were fullers and weavers, experts at the loom. They weren't Roman either.

Her father was. And once upon a time, he had lived in the town where he was employed by a large pottery, but since the death of his wife he had chosen to move to the village because he wanted to raise his daughter there.

And so she watched the men working the fields, hoeing, planting, scything, or driving sheep down the road, shearing and cleaning fleeces in open pens. The women could be seen tending vegetables or winnowing, shuffling the threshed grain in baskets to separate out the chaff. None of this fitted with Aelia's fantasy. She had ambitions. She was going to marry a soldier, a true Roman like her father. He had told her about his motherland – the vineyards, olive trees and rich orchards – maybe she would go there one day. The soldiers went back when they'd completed their service.

According to her father, some Roman women lived the life of princesses. They wore extravagant clothes: their robes were edged with embroidery from magical islands called Elis and Ceos; their slippers were laced with gold; and they dabbed *tejpat* perfume behind their ears. Emeralds and sardonyxes glowed at their throats and on their fingers. Their breath smelled of cinnamon and they ate delicacies – wild thrushes caught in nets, peeled fruit, fish flavoured with spices. This was to be her life, she was certain of it. Perhaps her father would go with her. He could abandon his industry and return to Rome. When she'd fulfilled her duties as a wife, she would soothe his worn hands, the cracked nails ruined by glaze, and the skin shiny with the fresh memory of burns from the kiln. They would live in a villa, because her soldier-husband would be high-ranking. They might even have a servant. And there would certainly be children. Children were central to Aelia's dream, despite her mother's story. She'd decided years ago that the gods would be on her side.

*

Two bottles later and Suzy's mood has lightened. The pasta was pronounced delicious – *and that's official* – even Barney asked for more and they used seconds as a bribe, making him play Hearts before going back to his bedroom.

With Barney gone, Leo lights up. Cal fingers the cigarette packaging, circling the bull's-eye design with the tip of her finger. 'Why do you smoke Lucky Strike?'

'Because it makes me look good.'

'Ponce.'

'You can talk, Daniel. You're the one who refuses to buy clothes designed by anyone other than Armani or whoever happens to be *it*.'

'So? You're only young once.'

'Okay, guys. Enough already.' Cal is smiling at them. She's used to intervening.

Suzy enters the conversation from leftfield: 'Have you two ever thought about having kids?'

'Whoa. Where did that come from?' Dan rears away from the table in mock fear. There might as well be a tarantula on his plate.

'Oh, I don't know. Just something I've been thinking about recently. Because of my research actually. Lots of – ' She falters, aware of Cal's eyes on her. This isn't something they've talked about in depth, partly because of Barney and partly because between them they've got a career and a PhD to keep them occupied. And it hits Suzy – they've never talked seriously about having children together. And why would that change all of a sudden? She's getting older obviously – isn't everyone? – but she hardly needs to keep an eye on the biological clock. Not yet. So what is it? Perhaps she's right after all: that figurine has worked some kind of magic. She's under a spell. But that's silly. And she knows it's not the reason. She knows why she feels this way, and it's so painful she can't even bear to contemplate it right now.

Leo shifts in his seat, leaning towards her, his elbows wide apart on the table. 'I did it years ago, you know.' He hesitates. 'I wish I could say I don't regret it. At least the part I regret is not thinking harder about how I would feel having a child and not being in his or her life.'

'But you could have been.'

'No, we agreed I was to stay anonymous. Just a sperm donor.'

'But what if you *had* had the opportunity to be there? You know. Like communal parenting?'

'I'm still not convinced. Course it's a right royal pain in the arse. Not the joint parenting bit, which has to be tricky, but trying to get someone pregnant. It wasn't as simple as a quick hand-job then bingo! It took several bungled attempts. I blame it on the turkey baster personally. Low-grade kitchenware. To be honest, I was relieved when it finally happened. I mean things got pretty tense. Anyway, I was only eighteen. I thought I was doing my part, you know, making some sort of statement.'

'Have you ever seen the kid?'

'No. They live up north. It's one of the reasons I moved to London actually.'

'Shit. That must have been really hard.'

Another pause. 'I'm over it, but yes it was hard.'

Cal starts to stack plates. 'Gosh, this is getting a bit intense. I've just spent a day on the baby farm. That'd be enough to put anyone off.' She's not looking at Suzy, although Suzy wants her attention. *How unkind.* Then again, Suzy realises she shouldn't have said anything, not like that in front of Dan and Leo. But the question seemed to pop out, unfiltered. She's obviously been spending too long cooped up alone in the flat. It must be the heat sending her loco.

*

Now they could see the town houses perched on the outcrop of land; they were no longer a dark smudge on the horizon. The stone tower loomed larger. They had the mule with them. Her father's pots were strung over his withers, back and rump, and they rose and fell a few inches with each step. Together, they'd loaded him up, making sure to pack the pottery with straw before binding it in sacking. The creature plodded on, head hung low, ears laid flat. It was Aelia's job to tend to him during the journey, clicking him on and checking his hooves for stones. She was fond of him, his odour of crushed grass and the curious way he chewed, the rubbery lips and jaw seeming to rotate at half-speed.

A few hours later, they were in the square in the shadow of the tower, setting up their stall. They'd been shown to their place by an official. All around them were shops, their wooden shutters flung open. A butcher's and ironmonger's. The carpenter and cobbler. The open stalls sold less common ware. Here were visions of excess – amphorae filled with olive oil and wine, skeins of wool in several shades, patterned cloths and leather goods, round cheeses and pyramids of fruits and vegetables. The gods – Priapus and Diana – had been generous and summer's bounty was beyond expectation, in spite of late frosts in the spring. The square seemed huge to Aelia and she couldn't begin to comprehend the number of people there. Her father watched as she took it all in and he smiled. He reminded her that they had a lot to do. And she felt niggled by him, held back. There was so much she wanted to see. She requested some time to visit the other stalls. He wasn't sure. So reluctant. But her expression made it impossible for him to refuse. He let her go, instructing her not to stray too far.

She threaded her way between the tables. The traders made declarations and appeals to customers, their voices ringing out. She took no notice and aimed directly for the temple. There, she found what she was looking for. She was greeted by the stallholder, a small man with thinning hair and the same ruined nails as her father. The stranger smiled at her, a leer she thought, and she felt embarrassed, but she stood her ground and examined the tokens: mostly feet, legs and hands; some ears as delicate as shells; lots of eyes decorated with white, blue and brown paint. All were uniform. This man had obviously made tokens for some time. The quality of a token was not necessarily important, Aelia knew that, but people liked to make the effort. Asclepius, god of health, wouldn't settle for shoddy work. Also available were seated figures, women suckling babes – no use to Aelia. And they were very expensive; they'd been imported and the clay was different to that which Aelia's father used; much finer. No, there wasn't a token that she wanted, and even if there was, she wouldn't be able to pay for one. The few coins that they owned were safe in her father's purse and she would have to ask him first. Why hadn't she thought about cost?

She left the stall disappointed, and found herself walking down one of

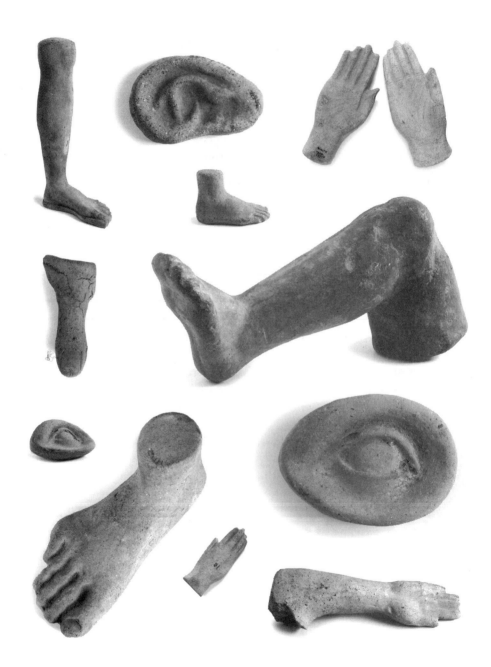

a network of narrow streets branching off the square. She was nosy, peeking into unshuttered rooms which were surprisingly small, despite the size of the buildings. Many of them were institutional – storage rooms or offices used by administrators. One street looked very much like another; there were no natural landmarks.

She stopped. Took a look around. How many streets had she turned down? She began to panic – she was disorientated – so she ran, head held high, watching the tower, hoping that it would guide her back to the square. Then she fell, tripping over a wooden crate, and found herself on her hands and knees. The street was covered in a layer of muck which oozed between her fingers and stained her tunic as far as the waist. She stood up and looked down at herself, then looked at the tower above the tiled buildings – it was so close, she could only be footsteps from her father's stall, and yet how would she get there? And what would she do about the mud? This day, the day that she had dreamt about for months, was suddenly so awful. Such an anti-climax. She was just a little girl, not a woman, no one had even noticed her, apart from the disgusting stallholder who had leered at her. And now she was alone in this strange place and she felt even more childlike. Tears began to roll, hot down her red cheeks. She abandoned herself to unhappiness, her shoulders heaving with sobs. But crying wasn't going to change anything; she'd have to ask someone for help.

*

Although it is the middle of the night, the heat in their room is stifling. Suzy can't lie still. Even with her legs scissoring the covers she feels hot and bothered.

'Cal, are you asleep? Caroline?' The humped figure next to her doesn't move.

'Please don't ignore me. I'm sorry, I just wasn't thinking. Too much wine.'

Cal tuts and shoves at her pillow. 'God, Suzy. Can't we just get some shut-eye? We'll talk about it properly tomorrow. In the not-so-cold light of day. My shift doesn't start 'til two.'

'Okay.'

Suzy gets out of bed and pads through rooms to the toilet. Lights go on and off one after the other in a domino effect. She returns, and gets close to her lover, fitting neatly against her back.

'Cal, I'm wide awake.'

Cal groans and fumbles in the dark for the switch to her bedside lamp. 'Okay, you win. We'll talk now. But this better be good.'

Suzy sits up and pulls the sheet around her, tucking it under her armpits. She flops her hands down onto her lap, weaving the fingers together, and then looks at Cal. Before she can say anything Cal starts the ball rolling. 'I can't imagine why you think I'd want to get pregnant again. You know how busy I am and a – '

'Hey, hang on. No, no, no! Who said anything about you having the baby? It's me. *I* want one. I have for ages, ever since – ' she stops, inhales. 'Ever since Mum died, you know. I want a family now that I haven't really got one any more, but I just haven't been able to admit it to myself. Or – or deal with it.' Her voice sounds strangled, and she slows down, trying to control her emotions. 'I've always known how hard it would be, especially because I could never just make a *mistake* and end up pregnant. You know what I mean? Some people just do it, don't they? Go out and get laid or whatever. But the thing is I feel so *broody*. It's driving me mad.'

Cal looks at Suzy in astonishment. 'You never struck me as the maternal sort at all.'

'But who does until their time comes? Anyway, you must still get it sometimes?'

'God! No.'

'But that's because you've got Barney, right?'

'Maybe, but that's different.'

'No it isn't. You've fulfilled a dream.'

'It wasn't like that, Suz. Not at all. I got pregnant because I thought it'd fix my marriage. I was in denial. And since I've done it – and 'cause of work of course – I think anyone who has romantic notions about having kids must be pie in the sky. Not that I don't love Barney. I do.'

'But you would have wanted kids, anyway. At some point.'

'I don't know. Look, Suzy, I can't help thinking this is about your work as well. You've reached the tough bit of your PhD. There's not enough going on.' She counters the dirty look that Suzy gives her and softens. 'I know how awful it's been for you, because of your Mum and everything. But that was over a year ago now. Have you spoken to your Dad about this?'

'Come on. He's the biggest emotional retard ever.'

'Suz! Look, you're frustrated. I can tell. And I get it. I do, really. You feel like you're missing out on something. I've got Barney and you want – '

'No! No. That sounds crazy. I'm not that pathetic, Cal. It's just that I never quite realised how much I want a baby till now. I need a family, my own children, child, you know. It's as simple as that. Just like everyone else. I want the security, and the fun too, and just because I'm gay, I don't see why I shouldn't be allowed to have that. Why is everything so hard and why do I sound so spoilt and babyish?' She's angry now, and still close to tears, but she can't help laughing at herself.

Cal rubs her eyes and lets out another groan, almost a growl, then takes Suzy in her arms. 'Oh sweetheart. You've really got to think hard about this. I mean, I worry about Barney. It hasn't started yet, the teasing, but when he's a couple of years older – well, I dread to think. It's hard enough for you and me, let alone bringing kids into the equation. My lot still flinch when I mention your name, for God's sake. You know what my brother's like.'

'I know. I know.'

'And anyhow, Suz, I mean you're so used to having all this time on your own and, let's face it, you're not exactly financially secure.'

'Okay, I know! I'm not thinking straight. It's *so* hot. Hang on.' And she gets up and opens the window wider and stands for a second, framed by the city sky at night tinted orange by light from the streetlamps. Then she turns back and crawls from the foot of the bed right up to Cal. She cups

Cal's chin in her hand and looks into her eyes. 'It's something I want us to do together, not just for me. *Our* baby. You know that I think Barney's fantastic. I love him. But I want my chance. Maybe not now. But when I've got a job and even maybe a bit of maternity leave. I know, it could be ages and everything but – '

'You better finish your goddamn PhD first. Then we'll talk about it seriously.'

'Yes, okay, okay. We'll get there, though. Let's say that much. Let's try and promise each other that we'll at least talk about it properly.'

'Okay. I promise.' Suzy kisses her now, and Cal returns the kiss before turning over. 'Right. That's it. I've *got* to sleep.'

*

Flavia Julius was exactly how Aelia imagined a Roman wife to be. Gentle, noble and unassuming. Aelia had spotted her through an open window; she had her back to Aelia, her plaited hair and elegant clothes illuminated in a rhomboid of sunlight. A woman, yes, a woman would help – and without wasting any time Aelia had banged on the door and rushed through an explanation when that door was opened.

But Aelia hadn't expected such kindness. Flavia introduced herself and invited Aelia into her home. Everything was neat and in its place – the glass jar and little brass lamps, a bowl of red apples and even a sculpture of the winged Victory. These were the details that Aelia noted, more novelties for her to take in and try to remember. There was a proper place to wash; Flavia had led Aelia there and helped her clean her hands. She even gave Aelia a freshly laundered *stola* and they'd left her coarse tunic to soak in salted water.

Flavia sat down and regarded the girl. There were questions she wanted to ask. Did Aelia's father know anything of her plans? Had she warned him about her desire to visit the temple? The girl bowed her head.

She hadn't known how to tell him. He was so kind, but he was nothing like a mother. He wouldn't have understood. Flavia paused to gather her thoughts. How old are you, she asked. Nearly sixteen, the girl told her, even though she had only just turned fifteen. Flavia commented that that was a fine age and Aelia blushed with pleasure. Flavia continued: she told Aelia how pretty she was. She would have her wedding ceremony. She would wear special robes with a woollen girdle and a chaplet of flowers in her hair. Her veil would be as bright as a sunrise and her shoes the colour of saffron. Flavia would help Aelia to explain how she felt to her father. And then, when the time came, Aelia would have her babies. Beautiful babies with soft hair and fat cheeks to pinch.

Flavia stopped speaking and smiled, absent-mindedly resting a hand on her huge belly, the belly that Aelia had been unable to take her eyes off. Flavia saw that she was being observed and invited the girl to rest her hand there too.

The girl moved to Flavia's side as she shifted in her creaking wicker chair, and she knelt before the older woman, raised a hand, and gently spread her fingers over the bump.

Aelia's eyes grew wider and she checked Flavia's face. She could feel the baby kicking hard. Didn't it hurt? Flavia laughed. It didn't hurt although it sometimes kept her awake at night. And she was certain it had to be a boy with a kick like that. Aelia agreed that Flavia would have a boy, then corrected herself. Lots of girls too, she added.

Flavia didn't mind. All she wanted was to have a healthy baby. Then she rose slowly from her chair, supporting her back. She told the girl to wring out her tunic and hang it in the sun to dry. Then they would make a visit to the temple before they went to find the girl's father. Aelia had said he was a potter. Flavia wanted to know more. So Aelia was a potter's daughter? Yes, the girl confirmed, puzzled. Flavia took her hand. 'Then you must do one thing for me. You must take a piece of clay and make a token, a woman my shape, a *matre*. Do the best you can. Put her in the kiln. Then find a pool, somewhere tranquil, somewhere the gods might visit, and throw in the figure. Say a prayer: wish for my baby to have a long life and offer your services to the mother goddess.'

Aelia looked into the eyes of her new friend. She made a promise to do so.

*

The next morning Suzy leaves Cal sleeping and goes into the kitchen, still cluttered with the debris of last night's meal. She washes her hands then dries them. She opens the larder cupboard and finds flour and a sachet of yeast there. She gets out the glazed mixing bowl and finds the scales, makes her measurement, then sifts the flour, letting it fall in drifts into the bowl. Pushing aside the dirty plates, grubby wine glasses and empty bottles, she flours the work surface. She adds hot water to the yeast in a measuring jug, then pours the liquid into a dimple in the mound of flour. Just as her mother once showed her, she starts to work the dough, shaping the mixture into a ball and moving it onto the worktop. She begins to knead, putting all her strength into the job, folding and kneading, and folding and kneading again.

Cal comes into the kitchen, yawning. 'Ugh. Give me coffee.' And she goes straight to the kettle and unplugs it. 'What are you up to?'

'It's a surprise. Do you fancy going on an adventure tomorrow?'

'Yeah, okay. Barney's going to his Dad's, so that'll be fine.'

'Great.'

Suzy wraps the dough in a chequered cloth and takes it to the airing cupboard where she leaves it in the dark to rise.

They are in the car heading for Cambridge. It's overcast, but the two women have still got the air-conditioning going full blast. There's a packet of jelly babies on the dash. Suzy takes one and offers the open bag to Cal who's at the wheel.

'You choose for me. Any colour.'

Suzy pulls out a purple one and holds it to Cal's mouth and Cal takes a bite, keeping her eyes on the road. 'Yum.'

'You went for the head first, you barbarian.'

'I couldn't see. I'm driving!'

'Poor excuse. I know your type.' Suzy feeds her the rest of the jelly baby before putting a tape in the stereo. Dolly Parton and John Denver. Cal loves Country and Western, in a cheesy kind of way, and they sing along in harmony.

Two hours later, Suzy instructs her to pull up.

'Why?'

'Just wait and see.' She's studying an OS map, turning it clockwise, then turning her head as a dog might cock its ear. 'This way.' Suzy gets out of the car and strides ahead. She has a striped carrier bag with her.

'Come on. It's not far.'

They walk through a copse, thick with nettles and brambles laden with fruit, although the berries are still tight. Sunshine is forcing its way through the cloud-cover, and shafts of watery light fall between trees. There's a path already made for them, not too obvious, but good enough to avoid nettle-stings and scratches.

'There!' Suzy strides ahead of Cal.

'What is it?'

'Come and look.'

They've arrived at an opening circled by common alder and yellow flag iris, the flowers like origami.

'Wow.' Cal moves towards the small pond, drawn to the still surface, glassy and dark. 'And – what?'

'It's a sacred pool,' Suzy explains.

'How do you know?'

Suzy looks heavenwards. 'I don't *know* for sure. I'm making an educated guess, that's all. One of the votive figurines, my favourite actually, was found not far from here with a horde of broken pot shards and a few coins. A local archaeological society organised a dig. The pond was probably larger then. That's what I reckon. The objects would have been thrown into the water. Part of a ritual, you know, with a prayer to a particular god, or a goddess in this case. Water had magical properties.'

'Well, it's very beautiful.'

Suzy takes something from her bag.

'What've you got there?' Cal peers over her shoulder.

'You don't half kill the moment sometimes, Cal.' Suzy hesitates then hands over the bread she made the previous day.

'My God. It's pregnant bread. Did you make her?'

'Yeah.' She eyes Cal, mildly offended. 'She's a bit crude, but you can tell it's a pregnant woman, can't you?'

'Just about.'

'Now make a wish.'

'What?'

'Make a wish or say a prayer or blessing. Whatever you want. Just in your head if you prefer.' She waits. 'You know what mine is.' They look at each other. 'Maybe not now, I know. But when the time's right.'

'Okay.' Cal sighs and closes her eyes.

'Now throw in the bread.'

Cal does as she's told and lobs the food sculpture into the pool. The bread smacks onto the water's surface without much dignity and finally, when it's sodden, it begins to sink, leaving behind a few grey bubbles. The last concentric rings lap at the pool's banks. Cal goes to Suzy, takes her hand and kisses her on the cheek.

'Thank you.' Suzy leans back, her face tilted to the sky diffused now with pale light. 'Isn't it amazing? I can't help loving this time of year.'

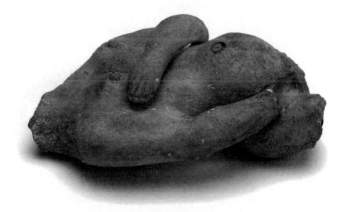

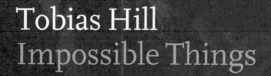

Tobias Hill
Impossible Things

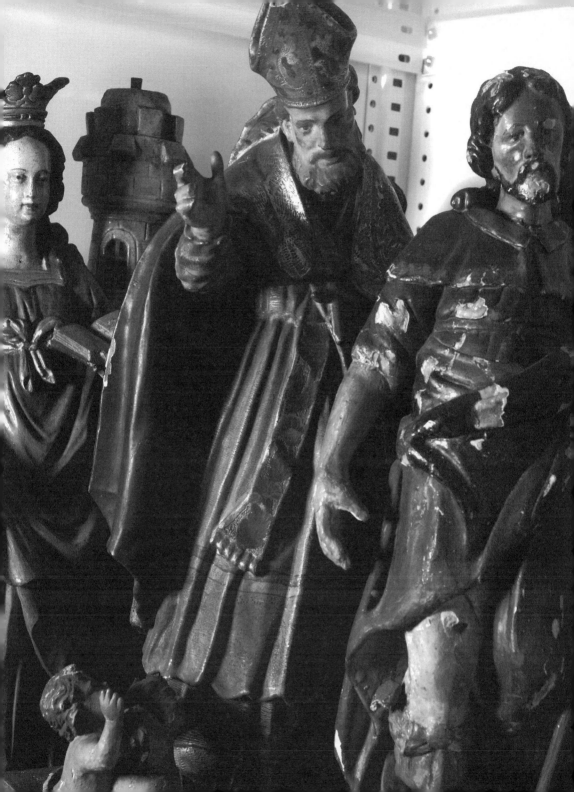

S OME PEOPLE HAVE A FEAR OF WATER. Peter has a fear of snow. It has something to do with the definition of space, the way the sky is abruptly revealed, huge, plotted out in the helter-skelter course of snowflakes. When it happens, it always occurs to him that the sky is much larger than he thought, and that he is smaller than he ever imagined.

Chionophobia: fear of snow. From the Greek, Peter thinks, and besides a moment of sharp envy – the thought of Mediterranean summers – he tends to leave it at that. There are certain limits to what he is prepared to consider about himself, and this phobia is one of them. It has been with him as long as he can remember, though the source of it is lost to him now, and he doesn't search himself for explanations. It is something he has almost never spoken of, in fact, not to his young wife, nor even to himself, alone; so that each time it happens it comes to him as something well forgotten. The sky moving above him, and the dread of it.

It is October. He is travelling on business, waiting on the quay at Dover. It is cold, he keeps his driving gloves on. He wears a Trilby, conveniently concealing his perennially advancing baldness; a bespoke suit, a coat of full chrome English leather.

The ferry is late. His head aches, as it has done intermittently since the war, the wound always at its worst in cold weather. Last Christmas his wife said he was like a bear with a thorn. He wonders how she puts up with him.

He looks up from *The Times* with an intimation that something is wrong. The sky, which has been dull all day, has darkened to the colour of old ironclads. Even as he watches, the first light flakes begin to fall.

If there is a worse omen for the journey he can't imagine it. Although he is suspicious of learning he is educated, nevertheless, and so it is the

Romans he thinks of, Caesar turning back from the Channel at the auguries found in the flight of birds. He is forty-two years old, a man who has made something of himself, but just for a moment, as the snow seesaws down onto the crowded quay, stippling the water, he is much younger again. His flesh shrinks under his skin.

He stands by the car, hunkered into his coat, while the ferry crowd grumbles and mills around him. His first urge is to turn back, but the traffic is a dozen vehicles deep behind his own. It is all he can do not to glance up. Instead he folds the newspaper, gets back into the Crossley and shuts the door behind him. In the shelter of the car he closes his eyes, squeezes them shut, praying that when he opens them the snow will have blown itself out.

He counts up to a hundred and back down to nothing. He opens his eyes. The sky outside has lightened perceptibly. The scattered flakes have already melted away on the windshield. Only the pinched faces of the second-class passengers waiting in the cold suggest it has ever snowed at all. Peter barks a short laugh, one part incredulity, two parts relief. What an odd thing, he thinks. It is only October, early for snow, but still it seems to him impossibly fortunate, the way his luck has turned and turned again. I am Alice's Red Queen, he thinks, with her six impossible things before breakfast. He wonders what the other five will be. Knowing the ferries, he is sure that breakfast will be one of them.

A car hoots further back in the queue. He starts the engine and edges forward all of a yard, switches it off, raises a hand good-naturedly to the disgruntled driver behind him.

There is still no sign of the ferry. On the seat beside him lie the discarded newspaper, his passport, and two logbooks; a company record, thick with carbon paper, and a smaller, personal diary. After a moment he picks up the second volume, takes a pen from his coat, and begins to write.

Captain Peter Johnston Johnston-Saint: this is the name on his passport. The document is genuine enough, the name less so. Only his aunts call him Percy now. His wife teases him over the assumed double-barrel. Elsewhere he is free to be the kind of man he has always dreamed

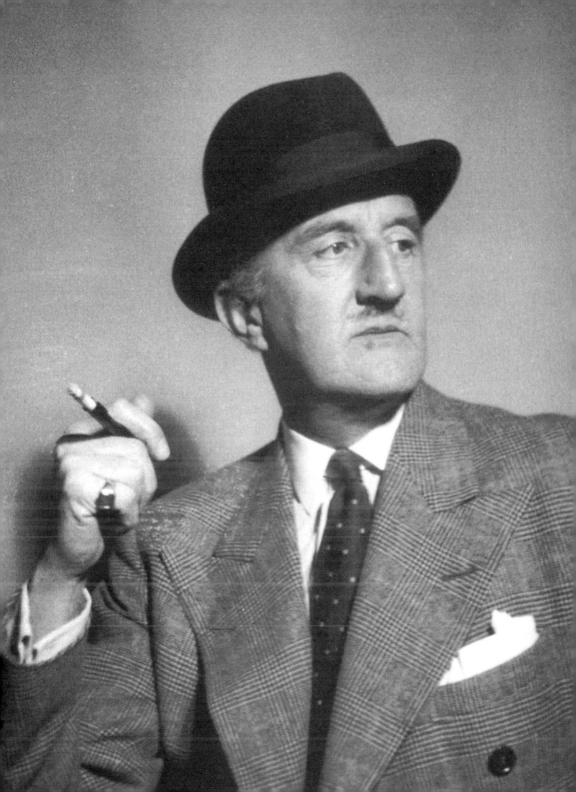

of: an officer and a polyglot, a driver of fast cars, a smoker of continental cigarettes, a lover of women. A husband. A man with a job worth talking about, too, as of this year; he is the European buyer for Henry Wellcome, *the* Wellcome, millionaire, international purveyor of medicines, eccentric collector of the history of the human body.

In his suitcase he carries a small fortune of Wellcome's money, six thousand pounds, one third in French francs. At times the transactions he undertakes are better made quickly, and the anonymity of cash is often as desired by the seller as the buyer. Wellcome himself is almost never mentioned. Peter knows he is a front, presentably less than wealthy, and is not offended by the idea.

In Paris, Berne, Lugano and Rome there will be additional funds waiting for him in a variety of currencies. If he were a certain type of individual he could disappear in any of these places, rich overnight, though he knows he never will. It is not a question of honesty. In Cairo a famous caricaturist once drew a sketch of him on the back of a postcard, and wrote underneath, *They call him Saint, but is he?* Peter would be the first to admit that he is less than that. It is not high morality that will bring him home in two months, so much as the need for a past, for the audience of those who know him.

He is forty-two years old. He wears his new names like tailored clothes. He does not think of himself as a vain man. The boyish part of him – not small, even now – imagines his work as a reflection of the best in him. It is like the life of a spy, he thinks, or a diplomat. Or a protagonist.

*

Mon. 15th Oct. 1928

8.15 am. Snow. If the weather gets no better I shall wait it out in Paris. Apparently also a collision in the Channel this morning. All ferries delayed till the last trump sounds over Dover. Docks crammed with bad-tempered drivers, women bristling in their new winter furs, foul-mouthed dogs frantic at the prospect of travel. *The Times* says dull weather, worse on the way. None of it has done much for my head nor my temper, but my spirits are high, considering.

Missing Clare. The first time out for Wellcome we made a holiday of it. C reading out Baedeker. Snippets like morsels from an Xmas hamper. We raced the South Eastern to the coast. London behind us. Ahead the cliffs, the sea & all beyond it.

I tell myself it is only two months and wonder if C does the same. The Crossley is as out of sorts as her master, needing attention I'll not have the time to give her today. Dover all bombsites and hoardings – I can't imagine what we saw in it. Drab streets hemmed in by the dubious claims of Vi-Spring Mattresses, Truphonic Hearing Aids, Henning's Patent Bending Machines. Modern clutter of stuff and promises.

Dirty Capitalism, the Leninists at Speaker's Corner call it. Clare took me to hear them once. They savour their words like preachers. No doubt they'd lump me in with the devil now if they knew what I do, and for whom.

How the devil are you? the gentlemen at the Aviatic will ask tonight; and *What are you doing with yourself, these days?* Well. I shall tell them that, these days, I'm in Stuff and Promises. Or I shall say, Acquisitions. Acquisitions has a better ring. I have been collecting for Henry Wellcome for three months now. It is fair to say that acquisitions are my business.

2.45 pm. Aboard at last. The ferry is a new design, a *ro-ro*. We drove on at one cavernous end and will trundle off the other at Boulogne, like so many sows herded to market. The squeal of metal and chains. As risibly ugly a mode of transport as I have ever seen in motion.

Clare would say it is early to be drinking. Clare would say, *No husband of mine needs to drink before noon.* But Clare is not here, only two salesmen in Harrods suits and a woman feeding vol-au-vents to a chow. Therefore I sit & write with whiskey and Perrier ticking at my elbow, like a timepiece.

This unseasonable weather does not agree with me. At least there is writing to be got on with. Writing has always done me good. It is better for the migraines than any of Wellcome's medical prescriptions (which I carry at his insistence. Packets labelled Lead with Opium, The Forced March, The Livingstone Rouser). A perk of the employment, the quantity of writing it will allow.

I should be working. I should write up the company log in triplicate. Army work ethic be damned – I do not have to jump to orders now. Tomorrow I am Wellcome's collector. There are men to see about death masks, anatomical publications, a collection of Roman circumcision knives. Appointments with the Count de Beaumont and His Excellency Mgr Maglione. I will visit M. Rotgé again. But for now I will have this little space to myself. My own log, for my own thoughts. There are still some things not even Wellcome can buy.

5.30 pm. The Aviatic, r. de Vaugirard. From the window the Tour Eiffel. Dusk gathering around it. A racket of trams. There are still street hawkers down there, hoping for one last sale.

The hotel is less well-kept than I remember it. The faded grandeur of the entrance, flanked with obelisks, busy as a Cairo bazaar. The Empire Suite Lounge, wreathed in the pall of cheap cigars. My rooms, too, are poky and cold. The bed is impossibly narrow.

Someone has left the Bible open at Esaïe. *Leur idoles d'argent et leurs idoles d'or, qu'ils s'étaient faites pour les adorer, aux rats et aux chauves-souris.*

Aunt Gwynne would look down her nose. Certainly these are not the lodgings she would choose; they are not of the best. *Your father would not have approved*, she would say. Little more than the choice of a successful travelling salesman, this place, which is not far off the mark, where I am concerned. I wonder whether my father would have approved of that either.

Dinner is served late here. I shall keep on my regimental tie. In the right circumstances it is better than a formal introduction. I must make the best of myself, for the sake of Henry Wellcome.

Settled down with the last of my Normandy guide. I have travelled with too little to read – the newspaper is finished, & Bible and lounge magazines besides there is nothing else here but Wellcome's medical guide (*For Explorers, Missionaries, Travellers, Colonists, Planters and Others*, one of which no doubt applies to me) and a pamphlet in green leather, for presentation only to the best company, outlining Wellcome's ambitions and aims:

> For many years I have been engaged in various researches respecting the early methods employed in the healing arts, both amongst civilised and uncivilised peoples. I anticipate that the historical exhibition of medical, chemical and pharmaceutical objects which I am organising, to be held in London shortly, will lead to the revealing of many facts, and the elucidation of many obscure points. Even though the items be ever so small, they may form important links in the chain of historical evidence...

Henry Solomon Wellcome. How the staff talk about him, as if he were nothing to be frightened of! The Old Man, they call him behind his back – though not too loudly, in case the walls hear. Then when he appears – unannounced, as often as not – they scurry like rabbits at the verge to be out of his way, or freeze under his stare. Like some mythological beast, they treat him. An old, shuffling monster. A notch-eared sphinx.

He is not so old. Older, perhaps, since his marriage foundered. I suppose he must be in his seventies, but with the energy of a younger man. Britchford says he was different before the separation. He says his collecting of all things medicinal was more of a diversion then, a rich man's hobby. Britchford says he talked of the museum with pleasure.

He does not do so now. Or if he does, the pleasure is too fierce. Quickly banked, as if it embarrasses him. The collecting is not a hobby now.

He talks to me. Apparently he likes me. We discuss the war, my travels, the diseases I have had. At my job interview he quizzed me about Rift Valley Fever until it was, frankly, embarrassing. He is on speaking terms with Britchford also. He is more comfortable with the workers among us, I think, the buyers and carpenters. It is the curators and the laboratory workers who propagate the myth that he never speaks. But he is a businessman who has made his fortune from medicine, not a medical man. An enthusiast, not a professional. I suspect that is how he sees it. It is how I might also see myself.

They say he was handsome once. Now he has the face of a mill-owner. Unapproachable dignity. It is rather hard to meet his eye. I find it impossible not to respect him. But I do not think I know him. I wonder who it is, these days, who does.

Tues. 16th Oct.

9.40 pm. To the Count, to make an appointment with Dr & Mme Sorrel-Déjerine re the Déjerine papers and apparatus. On to His Excellency in the Avenue du Président Wilson, with a view to an Audience in Rome.

I write this diary for an audience of one, therefore I will be honest with myself: since the war has left me with no qualifications besides four languages, a recurrent migraine and the ability to drive any model of car, it is likely on the basis of family contacts that I have my job. Not that there has been any intercession on my behalf. It is that I know who to approach, in Paris, Rome, Delhi, Dakkar. The Foreign Secretary, Wellcome calls me. He means it as a compliment, and I take it in that vein. I am the Ambassador of the Museum of Medicine.

From the Ave. du Wilson to Rotgé's by a roundabout way, but he was out. I would not bother myself with him again, except that Wellcome was so insistent. The shop looks shut up for good – is so fantastically decrepit, in fact, that the property almost certainly remains his. Cleared a space on the window to look inside. The floor is still laid with the pages of old books, paper and, here and there, ruined vellum. A pair of spectacles lay on the counter by a bottle of Ricard, a jug, a glass, all empty. He has not gone far. I will be back for him.

pm to M. Boulanger. Last month he sent a catalogue to us – never a promising sign for business. A mare's nest of a collection. Eye-baths in bottle-green, blue, white: red-beaded, tasselled Incan medicine caps sprawled on their shelves like crustacea. A battered selection of prosthetic hands and hooks in wood, steel and whalebone. A treatise on fifteenth-century Welsh medicine, which I might have taken had it not been so damaged by mould (*To Extract a Tooth Without a Pin, take Newts, by some called lizards, and those nasty beetles which are found in ferns in the summer. Calcine them in an iron pot, and make a powder thereof. Wet the forefinger of the right hand, and insert it in the powder...*).

Also some tolerable pornography. Many of the ukiyo-e we have already. From £500 we meandered down to £450, by which time it was late and we were both tired of the whole business. Shook on it and extricated myself from the unexpected offer of a meal. A sullen man, and expensive.

All in all a full day's work. As reward I walked home along the river and didn't stop at a single stall. Weather here much the same as London. The sky is threatening.

Now I am back. The fire has been lit. The room is more welcoming than I could have imagined. The hatchet-faced maid has even brought my supper. Warm bread, cold cuts, red wine. I am missing Clare less – is this good or bad of me? Good or bad for me? Tonight I am at home with myself.

Weds. 17th Oct.

6.12 pm. Last night slept badly. Two dreams. The first was the old one in which I am young: I am not yet living with my aunts. I stand on tiptoe to peer out of a bedroom window – not mine. The world outside is thick with snow – the hills and trees turned white overnight, as if they have seen ghosts.

The second dream was new, and of Wellcome's warehouse. Willesden, the smell of railways and the Burgess Anchovy Essence factory. The miles of shelves where the bulk of the collection is housed. Overburdened, overshadowed aisles, already beyond all the ingenuity of the curators. Crates straining to split open.

Britchford says the backlog of unsorted material already goes back six years, and will only get worse. The warehouse staff work like sorcerer's apprentices. How many of us dream of Wellcome's dream, I wonder, as we go about our duties? As if, through our employment, he has bought us, just as he buys everything else.

Wellcome's ambitions overwhelm the lives of those around him. My own possessions, like my own ambitions, seem slight beside his. Even this diary of mine is small, bound in cheap nigger leather.

Rouen today, for a private library sale. Rain spitting as I set out. Passed several Delages on the road, a Whippet driving like a dirt-track racer, and next year's Lagonda Coupé, straight out of the show-room and already caked from boot to bonnet in honest Normandy mud.

The château was in a poor way. The roof, as the owner said more than once, cannot be patched with vellum. The family is short of money, but set on avoiding the publicity of an auction, even if it means they make a thinner profit. We agreed at £850 for the lot, less ten per cent for prompt cash payment.

pm, to the Monet collection in Rouen. I stayed later than I intended. They are certainly beautiful, though not quite to my taste. When the curator came to bustle me out I was only a third-way through the 30 views of Paris. All are the same and each is different. It is as if there are no facts of which anyone should be confident, only this endless process of light and time.

'What is the purpose of this collection?' I asked Wellcome at my interview, when he asked me for my thoughts. At the time it was a token question – my interest was rather less than genuine. And he said – his accent American but dulled like old pennies – 'Sir, I aim to collect together the complete history of human medicine.' Now I understand it was only half an answer. He said it without a smile, without any kind of pleasure at all, as if he expected me to laugh. I doubt anyone laughs at him to his face.

It sounded like a straightforward thing to find then, the history of medicine. It has taken me these last months to realise how many kinds of medicine there are. Wellcome no more collects one history than there is one Paris in the paintings of Monet.

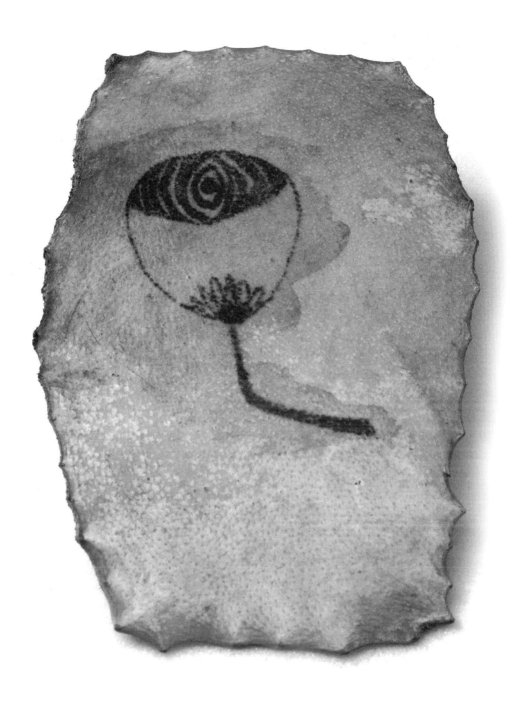

There are the categories of objects which would be acceptable in any public museum – the dry papers of eminent doctors, the dull instruments of dead surgeons. Then there are the possessions of those who are not doctors, as such, but who are said to wield medical power all the same. There are the failures of one medicine or the other, the preserved inoperable curiosities. There are the talismans, the evidence of miracles, the fetishes of twisted hair. The statues of the saints of birth pains, their feet worn smooth by the fingers of believers, the biological icons of erotica, the charms for afflictions of the heart, and the ritual knife in grey shagreen, and the craw-stones of crocodiles. There are men, those like Rotgé, who buy and sell such things.

On my last visit it was tattoos. Not plans, but the illustrations themselves. Rough lengths and flaps of skin, discoloured with hair and *acne vulgaris*, poorly preserved in surgical spirit. The illustrations themselves – of women, flowers, men-at-arms – were unexpectedly beautiful. They were old, Rotgé insisted, handed down and sold on by the family of a surgeon in the Napoleonic wars. Rotgé brought them up from his damp cellars and laid them out on that counter of his, next to his lunch and water glass. He handled them as a tailor would good silk.

'The exhibition will be strictly professional and scientific in character, and will not be open to the general public.' So Wellcome writes in his green leather book. When I brought the tattoos back to London, we talked about how they might be classified – should it be Section Two – Manuscripts – or Four (Medals, Emblems and Charms)? Section Five (Curiosities of Surgery) or Thirteen (Criminology)?

Tomorrow I will see Rotgé again. Wellcome has asked me to do so, but I will be honest with myself. I do not need his excuse. Such an ordinary man, with such impossible things.

*

He has been knocking for several minutes before anyone answers. The woman who opens the door is not the one Peter remembers, though she is similar in her reddish hair and the wary way she holds herself. He had assumed the first woman was Rotgé's wife, and now wonders if all three are relations of some kind.

He begins to explain himself. His voice in French is lower than in English, the tone less dynamic, more sanguine, as if language makes him a different man. Before he is done the woman has turned away, waving him in, calling a name – *Jean!* – to which there is no audible reply.

For a moment they wait together. The woman calls the name again, tapping her fingers on the shop counter, where the bottle, glass and jug still sit, opaque with days of dust: only the spectacles are gone.

'Jean!' The woman calls for a third time. She makes a sound – an impatient, oddly jubilant exhalation, like the cough someone will make after slaking a thirst – then leaves Peter without another word. There is the slam of a door, shouting, a man's voice replying dismissively – Peter catches only the word *vache* – then a barrage of French which leaves him rapidly lost. Almost as quickly the door to the back of the shop opens and Rotgé comes bustling in, rubbing his hands together. His fingers are black with earth. The smell of it permeates the small room.

'I am busy. What do you want?' he begins in French. 'Oh, it's you,' he adds in English, and Peter is thankful when he does not hold out his hand in welcome, but only takes the pipe out of his mouth. 'Why did you not say so? I was not expecting you.'

The woman appears at the doorway. For once Peter is not glad of the audience. He puts his hands in his pockets, searches for something to say. 'You were gardening?'

'Gardening,' Rotgé says. When he smiles his front teeth peek through his moustache. 'Of course. Perhaps I was digging for carrots.' His expression suggests he has made a joke. Peter tries not to think what it could be. 'Do you like carrots, Mister Saint?'

'Yes,' Peter says. 'As a matter of fact I do.' Rotgé nods, points with his pipe.

'Later my wife will cook for you. She is an excellent cook.'

'That would be very kind of her.'

'Of course. Her food will make you well. Food is the medicine of the peasant. Are you sick, Mister Saint?'

'No, I am quite well. Thank you.'

'But you have not heard this saying? That food is the peasant's medicine?' He answers without thinking. 'Never.'

'Still, perhaps your employer would like to buy some of my carrots?'

'No, sir, he would not.' He is irritated to hear his own terseness. Rotgé's grin relaxes into a more comfortable smile. He leans back against the shop counter.

'Then I am mistaken. I understood that your Mister Wellcome was looking for medicine. I have been told that he will buy every curative his representatives can find. He is a rich man, is he not? A transatlantic American. Such an interesting, a curious ambition. Perhaps it is he who is unwell? My wife has a special recipe –'

'I am not here for your carrots, sir.'

Silence falls between them like a blade. In the doorway the woman edges from foot to foot. Peter clenches his hands in his pockets and looks nowhere. The identity of his employer has never been discussed; it is news to him that Rotgé knows even his name. He wonders if this is the point of the man's joke, and finds that he would be relieved if it was.

'So,' Rotgé shrugs. No longer smiling, he has become abruptly, enthusiastically professional. 'Then we will do business. Please, sit down,' he says, and frowns – there is nowhere to sit. Without looking at the woman in the doorway he speaks again in French, low and venomous, and she leaves and reappears almost immediately, dragging two chairs, each almost as large as herself. Rotgé waits until she is gone before repeating his offer. 'Sit, Mister Saint. Please.'

They sit. A clock ticks unevenly, somewhere in an adjoining room. It is still early. Peter glances at the window: outside the morning has brightened. Light filters through the dirty panes where he peered in two days ago.

When he looks back Rotgé is relighting his pipe. His fingers are clenched around the burr stem, the dirt under his nails black as old blood. Out of nothing Peter thinks of the drive back from the château near Rouen. A country road, sunk between fields of marl and limestone.

'In fact, it is good to see you again.' Rotgé waves the match out. 'Business has been unkind to me. My circumstances have worsened, as you can tell,' he says, motioning apologetically at the half-abandoned shop. Peter nods, less than honestly, as if he remembers Rotgé in kinder times.

'I knew you would come back, of course.'

'Really?'

'Of course! Because, you see, I know who you work for. This wealthy Mister Wellcome – he has become quite famous in some places. Everyone would like to do business with the famous Mister Wellcome. Even you are becoming a famous face!' Rotgé's own face lights up. 'The Englishman who drives fast cars, eh? Well, and so I know I will see you again. There are things you will not find for your Wellcome in just any pharmacy. You must come back to your old friend – Rotgé.'

He has begun to smile again. There is an anxiety to the expression that Peter cannot help but find faintly repulsive. Rotgé draws on the pipe and leans forward. 'I have even kept something for you. A special purchase.'

'How kind of you,' Peter says, and Rotgé's eyebrows rise, as if with suppressed laughter.

'You will see! You will see I have found what you are looking for!'

*

It is nothing at all. A squat box and raised cylinder of polished wood and brass, a maker's plate on the back. A resinous excretion encases one side of the apparatus. An inductor coil, Peter thinks. It is no different from countless other old medical curios that he has purchased or passed over in the markets of a dozen cities during his work for Wellcome.

'What do we have here?' he says, and Rotgé laughs, a little uneasily. He has been wearing worn felt gloves, and he takes them off quickly now, crumpling them into the pocket of his coat.

'Just as you see.'

'It looks like an inductor.'

'Exactly. An inductor coil. Made by the firm of Eugène Ducretet, in Paris, in the last decade of the last century.'

'Well.' He makes a half-hearted attempt to hide his bewilderment. It is something he feels personally, an acute sense of anticlimax. The lack of the impossible.

'You are disappointed.'

'No, no.'

'This is not the kind of thing you are looking for.'

'It is exactly the kind of thing,' Peter says, and almost adds, But it is not the kind of thing I expected from you.

'You must tell me,' Rotgé says, insistently smiling, goading, almost, 'if you are disappointed,' and this time Peter finds himself at a loss to do anything but tell the truth.

'Yes,' he says. 'Well, if you must know. From the hullaballoo you gave it, I expected something a little more...'

'It is alive.'

'I'm sorry?'

'It is alive,' the merchant says again, as if he is pointing out the obvious. The weather outside, the price of a dish on a printed sheet. Peter bites back the urge to laugh.

'Is it?'

'I am told so, yes. People say it is living, and that it will cure the one who owns it.'

'Cure him of what, exactly?'

'Of many things,' Rotgé says, and reaching into his pocket he hands Peter the felt gloves.

He stands without meeting Rotgé's eye, embarrassed for him. Instead he looks at the apparatus. Beyond his first cursory glance he has barely considered the thing itself. Now he puts on Rotgé's gloves and does so.

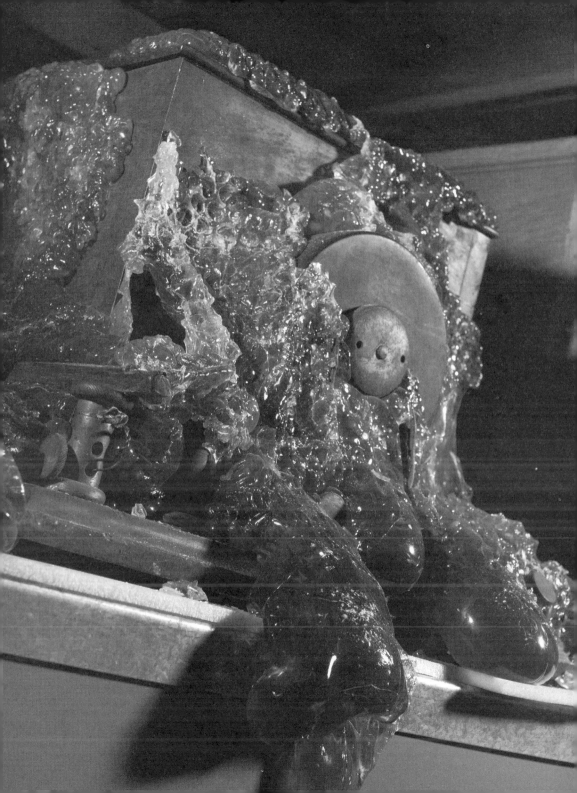

others a figure of Santa Appolonia. I enquired about a photograph but none was to be had.

Burjasot and Albufera.

In the afternoon I took a car to the outlying villages of Burjasot and Albufera where I obtained from the villagers some interesting samples of herbs used by the local inhabitants for various purposes.

Bookshop of Manuel Berenguer Molera.

On my return to Valencia in the evening I called in with my guide at an old book shop which might be described for want of a better word as a junk shop of the first order. It was in a narrow dirty street and it was lighted by one gas jet. The proprietor was reclining in a broken wicker chair smoking the stump of a cigar. All around him in the small room, some 12' x 10' were piles of books - the floor was a mass of rubbish, loose leaves, pamphlets, vellum bound books and such like which you had to walk on indiscriminately. Nevertheless he produced some unique medical books on Spanish Medicine. Most of these books were of the 16th and 17th Century and are extremely hard to obtain in Spain. The proprietor told me that "Maggbross" of London bought many books from him. I knew whom he meant though it was difficult to recognise from the pronunciation. Amongst these books was one dated 1547 in old Gothic characters on Magic and Superstitions, in Spanish. The proprietor, Manuel Berenguer Molera, Poeta Querol, 10, Valencia, told me that "Maggbross" had written him several times asking him to send these books off to him, but that he had been so busy that he had not had the time!! I purchased the last batch of these books from him for £20 and also the book on Magic for £6. There are about 150 books in all.

This arrangement took me up till 9 p.m. and as there was nothing further of interest in Valencia, I resolved to leave for Barcelona the following day.

A stillness falls on the room. There is absolutely nothing remarkable about the machine, Peter thinks, except for the substance it exudes. He does not touch either the coil or its excretion. From the back room or the cellar Rotgé has brought out a small, solid folding table, on which he has carefully placed the apparatus. The excretion covers one side of the box itself, then extends almost a foot below its case. Rotgé has arranged it in such a way that the stuff hangs over the lip of the table. It has the colour and translucency of honey, or something richer, the resin of trees he has seen tapped in warmer climes. It would be almost beautiful, Peter thinks, if it were not for its skin.

The surface of the substance is not smooth, as his experience suggests it should be. Instead it has grown a pattern, a network of approximate but well-defined hexagons. Some of the cells have closed in on themselves, like blisters. Like the combs of bees, he thinks, and the idea brings him up instinctively, stops him touching, sits him back in his chair.

'This substance is a chemical reaction?'

'Perhaps.'

'You think not?'

'I am told it is not.'

'Do you always believe what you are told?'

'No.' Rotgé shrugs. He is smiling again, as if the pleasure has not yet gone out of the transaction. 'My wife's priest tells me that prayer will heal all ills. I do not believe him, but what does it matter? If your employer wishes to buy all cures, then he must buy all our prayers.'

'Yes, but this is a machine, Monsieur, not some religious relic –'

'You must buy many things for this history of medicine. Not only medicines. You must buy all the things that people put their belief in. The relics, yes, the statues of saints, the talismans,' Rotgé says. 'I have heard that you buy these things.'

'Well then.' Peter returns the smile with some force. 'Then you expect me to believe that this is something people put faith in. Is that it? But I have no proof that this is anything other than an interesting piece of medical equipment, and in rather less than fair condition. Why on earth should I believe it is anything more?'

'So. It is a mystery.'

They sit one on each side of the table, the apparatus between them like a game of chess. Rotgé is no longer smiling; he looks tense now, a merchant anxious not to lose a sale. Peter wonders why the man would have bothered with such a story. Perhaps he has lost his sources, whoever they are, he thinks; perhaps he has nothing else to sell. Still it seems strange. The thought kindles a spark of curiosity, and he puffs out his cheeks, as if he could blow it out.

'You don't touch it with your hands.'

'No.'

'You consider it dangerous? Is it poisonous?'

'No. I do not touch it because I have nothing to cure.'

'Well,' Peter begins. Part of him – the part that dislikes Rotgé – is glad of the rejection he knows he is about to make. But part of him is not; the disappointment on his face is real. 'I am very sorry. I am not prepared to buy this story, and I am certainly not about to spend my employer's money on this apparatus, whatever else it may be. I had hoped for better than this.'

Rotgé shifts forward in his chair, anxiously, as if he will say something at last, then sits back with an expression of failure. As if it is beyond him. 'Monsieur Rotgé,' Peter says, rising again from his chair, 'Thank you for the opportunity. I am afraid it is not quite –'

'I have kept it for you, Mister Saint. Especially for you. You will make a mistake,' Rotgé says, low and quick, almost angry, 'Such a mistake, if you do not take this.'

'Monsieur Rotgé –'

'I will not offer it to you again. I will not keep it for you.'

'I can see that it would be –'

'Take it, Mister Saint.'

'I will do nothing of the kind.'

'Take it. Offer me a price.'

'I will not.'

'Any price.'

'Why?' Peter says. And then, almost despite himself, the merchant in him still curious, still hoping for miracles, 'Any price, you say?'

Rotgé smiles. 'You will find that it cures many things.'

*

Paris, Rouen, Lugano, Rome. A leech-vase of red Roman glass, a pair of Foucault's spectacles, a foetal skull carved from bird bone. From Monsieur Nachet, a copy of Pasteur's *Maladies of the Silkworm*. From Madame Hirschbrunner, a small collection of instruments of torture. In the Vatican a ring to kiss. Room after room of cardinals.

He writes all of it down, recording it in triplicate for Wellcome, once for himself. The writing does him good, he thinks. At the very least it means he forgets nothing. For years afterwards he remembers the journey, every detail of it. But it is only the apparatus he dreams of.

It always begins with the same thing; the nightmare of Wellcome's collection. He is there in the warehouse, with the smell of railways and factories. In the last of the long aisles, just out of sight, Rotgé's machine waits to be unpacked again. He has been looking for it forever, it seems, but no one can ever find it.

The cargo crate creaks at the seams. In Peter's dream it never splits open. He never knows what lies inside, or whether it is dead or alive. There is only the sound of its pressure, the groan of rooms cracking at the keystones, the rooms of Wellcome's Museum filling as fast as they can be built. The past overtaking the present as the dead outweigh the living.

On December the sixteenth he leaves Paris for home. It is 1928, a cold winter. When he steps to the quay at Dover his wife is waiting for him. Clare, he says, and she just smiles and smiles. There is snow in her hair and on the collar of her fur and he draws it off and holds it for a moment, amazed, pressing it in his hand. As if it could warm him.

Wellcome's Things

These are the catalogued facts about the Wellcome collection objects featured in this book.

Abbreviations: SM – held by the Science Museum, Wellcome Library photograph; SSPL – held by the Science Museum, Science & Society Picture Library photograph; WL – held by the Wellcome Library, Wellcome Library photograph.

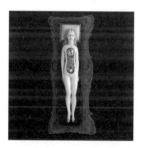 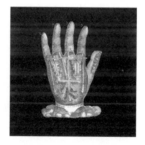

[Front cover]
Ivory anatomical model of a pregnant female with removable internal organs, on a cloth covered wooden couch with ivory pillow. Probably German, c. seventeenth century. SM, A127699

[Back cover]
Woodcut illustration of an artificial hand from Ambroise Paré's *Instrumenta chyrurgiae et icones anathomicae* (Surgical instruments and anatomical illustrations), Paris, 1564. WL, EPB 4818/B

'Body Art' by A. S. Byatt

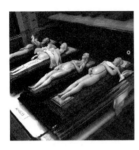 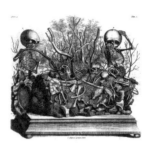 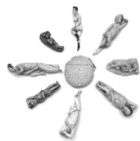

p. 1
Seventeenth and eighteenth
century ivory anatomical
models with removable
internal organs in the Science
Museum's Anatomy and
Pathology storeroom. WL

p. 2
Line engraving by Cornelius
Huyberts, 1709. A plate to
Frederick Ruysch's *Thesaurus
anatomicus octavus*,
Amsterdam, 1709. Ruysch, a
Dutch anatomist and pioneer
in techniques of preserving
organs and tissue,
constructed tableaux such as
this from body parts
including foetal skeletons,
gallstones and kidneystones,
veins and arteries. The actual
foetuses shown here are now
in the Academy of Sciences,
St Petersburg. WL, icon.
Anat. 202

p. 43
Eighteenth- to early
nineteenth-century
diagnostic dolls, used by
women patients to indicate
areas of affliction to their
doctors. Clockwise from top:
Ivory, Japanese. SM,
A641829;
Ivory, Chinese. SM, A626441;
White jade, Chinese. SM,
A78789;
Ivory, Japanese. SM,
A190390;
Ivory, Chinese. SM, A164587;
Ivory, Japanese. SM, A105357;
Ivory, Chinese. SM, A89122;
Ivory, Japanese. SM, A105356

At centre: Contraceptive
cellulose sponge, 'Clinocap'
brand. English. SM, A626871

'The Collected' by Hari Kunzru

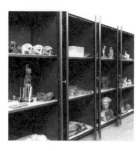

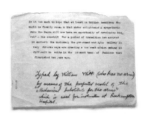

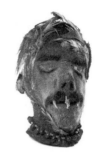

pp. 44–5
Bones and anatomical models in the Science Museum's Anatomy and Pathology storeroom. WL

p. 51
Slip of paper, typed by William Witt, from a notebook of writing practice which accompanied Mr George Thomson's 'Mechanical Substitute for the Arms'. Scottish, 1919. SM, A602321

pp. 54, 57
A shrunken head (tsantsa). Ecuador/Peru border, late nineteenth/early twentieth century. SM, A102935

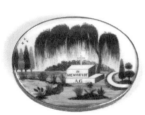

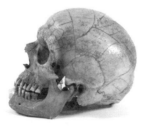

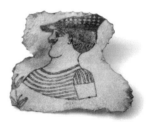

p. 61
Memento mori brooch containing a graveyard scene made from hair. Acquired before 1936. SM, A642442

p. 63
Skull inscribed in French with phrenological markings. One half shows the head according to the system of Gall, the other half according to that of his colleague, Spurzheim. European, nineteenth century. SM, A25407

p. 71
Human skin tattooed with a male bust and flower stem. French, 1850–1900. SM, A680

'Phantom Limbs' by Gaby Wood

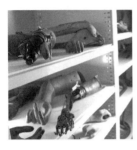

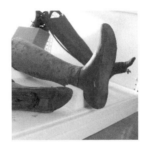

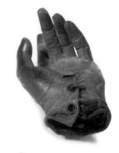

pp. 74–5
Artificial arms in the Science
Museum's Orthopaedics
storeroom. WL

p. 76
Artificial legs in the Science
Museum's Orthopaedics
storeroom. WL

p. 78
Wooden hand with brass wrist
plate and leather glove. The
fingers and thumb are
moveable. European,
1880–1920. SM, A653506

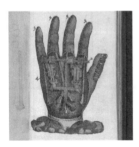

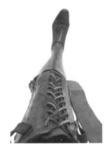

p. 81
Woodcut illustration of an
artificial hand from Ambroise
Paré's *Instrumenta chyrurgiae
et icones anathomicae*
(Surgical instruments and
anatomical illustrations),
Paris, 1564. WL, EPB 4818/B

p. 84
Artificial lower leg with laced
leather thigh socket. Made by
W. R. Grossmith for
amputation at the knee.
English, 1861–1920. SM,
A603149

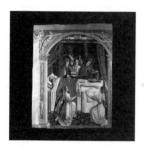
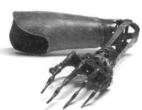
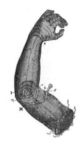

p. 87
Saints Cosmas and Damian
performing a miraculous
feat of surgery: amputating
the ulcerated leg of a
Christian and transplanting
in its place the undiseased
leg of a dead Moor. Oil
painting on panel, 168 x 133
cm. Attributed to the Master
of Los Balbases, Burgos,
Spain, c. 1495. WL, 46009i

p. 91
Steel hand and forearm with
brass wrist mountings and
leather upper arm socket.
European, c. 1890. SM,
A602817

p. 94
Woodcut illustration of an
artificial arm from
Ambroise Paré's *Instrumenta
chyrurgiae et icones
anathomicae* (Surgical
instruments and anatomical
illustrations), Paris, 1564.
WL, EPB 4818/B

'Milk' by Peter Blegvad

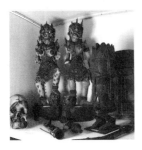

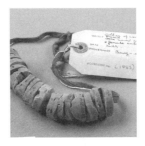

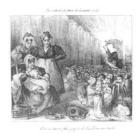

pp. 104–5
Shelf of objects in the Science Museum's Ethnography storeroom. WL

p. 109
Bootlace threaded with corks, placed around the necks of female cats or bitches to drain away milk. Boring-sur-Gironde, France, 1871–1920. SM, A666083

p. 112
Babies at a maternity hospital refusing to breast feed until the Houses (of Parliament) are dissolved. Coloured lithograph by J. E. Chaponniere, Paris. WL, 17491i

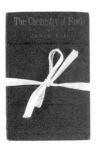

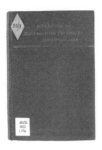

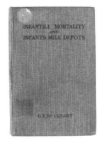

p. 114
The Chemistry of Foods: with microscopic illustrations by James Bell. London, published for the Committee of Council on Education by Chapman and Hall, 1881–3. WL, QU50 1881B43c Pt. 1

p. 114
Analysis of Milk and Milk Products by Henry Leffmann and William Beam. Philadelphia, P. Blakiston, 1893. WL, WA695 1893L49a

p. 114
Infantile Mortality and Infants [sic] Milk Depots by G. F. McCleary. London, P. S. King & Son, 1905. WL, XWA

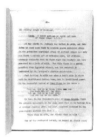

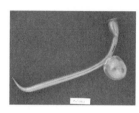

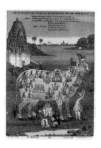

p. 118
'Some Notes on the History of
Milk' by A. W. Harris. A
hand-typed manuscript. WL

p. 119
Glass breast reliever. SM,
A606860

p. 120
The holy Cow personified as
World Mother with many
Sanskrit verses.
Chromolithograph. Bombay,
Anant Shivaji Desai Motibazar
Mumbai (Karla Lonavla: Ravi
Varma Press). WL, 26687i

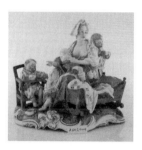

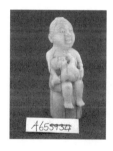

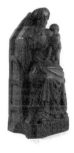

p. 125
Porcelain figure group of a
woman with two children,
breast feeding a baby,
possibly Frankenthal,
Germany, possibly 1755–99.
SM, A642949

p. 125
Small ivory effigy of mother
and child, woman sitting
down holding baby who is
being breastfed. Democratic
Republic of Congo,
1860–1910. SM, A655934

p. 125
Wooden figure of the Virgin
Mary as our Lady of
Tregurun, invoked by
mothers desiring to obtain
their milk, French,
1500–1600. SM, A75558

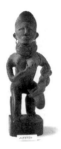

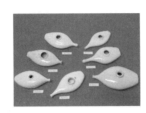

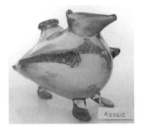

p. 126
Carved wooden figurine of
kneeling woman holding a
small child on one knee, other
hand clutching her left breast.
Padded cloth neckband.
Mayombo people, Democratic
Republic of Congo,
1880–1925. SM, A655930

p. 127
Seven boat-shaped infants'
feeding bottles, English,
1701–1900. SM, A625718,
A625725, A625723, A625522,
A625719, A625721, A 625724

p. 127
Glass infant's feeding bottle
in shape of bird with three
legs. Persian, eighteenth
century. SM, A85612

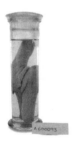

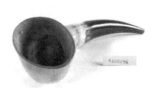

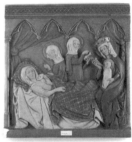

p. 127
Preserved calves' teats. Used
on infant feeding bottles
(before rubber). SM,
A600093

p. 127
Cow's horn used for infant
feeding, eighteenth century.
SM, A600088

p. 128
Plaster plaque showing a
scene of infant feeding by
Jane Jackson. Copied from a
thirteenth-century
manuscript, c. 1930. SM,
A651630

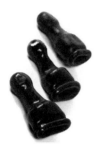

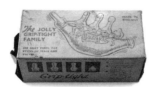

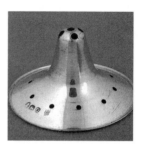

p. 128
Rubber teats made by Maw,
London, c. 1930. SM,
A625760, A632238pt1,
A632238pt2

p. 129
Glass infant's feeding bottle
in original box (the Grip-tight
miniature feeder) made by
Lewis Woolf Ltd,
Birmingham, c. 1935. SM,
A625800

p. 129
Silver nipple shield, 1811. SM,
A600098

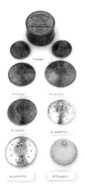

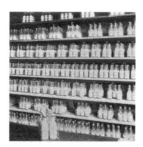

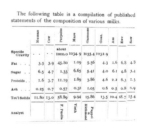

p. 129
Silver and celluloid nipple
shields. The two at the top are
sitting next to their original
box. English, nineteenth
century. SM, A606841,
A641268, A641257,
A600096, A641258,
A600098, A500007

p. 131
Illustration of the distributing
room of an infants' milk
depot in Battersea, London.
Taken from *Infantile
Mortality and Infants* [sic] *Milk
Depots* by G. F. McCleary.
London, P. S. King & son,
1905. WL, XWA

p. 131
Table showing 'statements
on the composition of
various milks'. Taken from
*Analysis of Milk and Milk
Products* by Henry Leffmann
and William Beam.
Philadelphia, P. Blakiston,
1893. WL, WA695 1893L49a

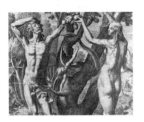

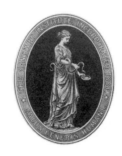

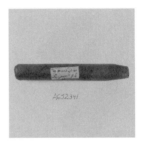

p. 133
A woman-serpent bends
around the Tree of Knowledge
as Adam and Eve reach into
the branches. Line engraving
by T. De Bry (1528–98) after J.
Van Winghe (1544–1603).
WL, 15624i

p. 134
Plate from the inside front
cover of *Analysis of Milk and
Milk Products* by Henry
Leffmann and William Beam.
Philadelphia, P.Blakiston,
1893. WL, WA695 1893L49a

p. 134
Length of bamboo, apparently
used as feeding tube for giving
milk to snakes, probably from
the Middle East, probably
second half of the nineteenth
century. SM, A652341

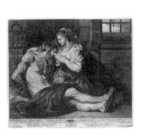

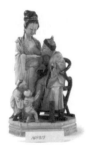

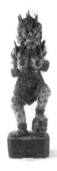

p. 138
Pero breast-feeding her
imprisoned father Cimon.
Line engraving by C. van
Caukercken (1625–80) after
P. P. Rubens (1577–1640).
WL, 18149i

p. 139
Ivory statuette showing a
woman breast-feeding her old
mother-in-law, watched by
her two children. Chinese.
SM, A69819

p. 140
Painted wooden figure of
female bare-breasted demon.
Polychrome with tongues of
flame issuing from the head
and shoulders. Carved in one
piece. From Lombok Island,
Indonesia, 1801–1900. SM,
A54516

'The Venus Time of Year' by Helen Cleary

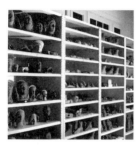

pp. 142–3
Graeco-Roman votive
offerings in the Science
Museum's Classical and
Mediaeval Medicine
storeroom. WL

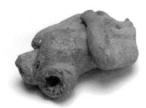

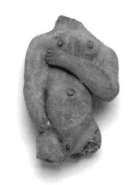

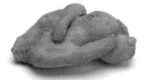

pp. 144, 149, 167
Votive pregnant female
figure, torso only, terracotta,
said to have been found in
Suffolk, Roman,
100BC–AD200. SSPL,
A634992

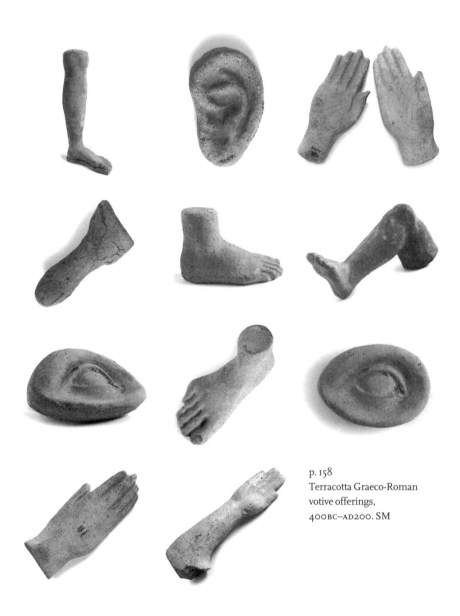

p. 158
Terracotta Graeco-Roman
votive offerings,
400BC–AD200. SM

'Impossible Things' by Tobias Hill

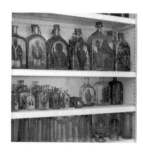

pp. 168–9
Holy water bottles in the
Science Museum's Medical
Glassware storeroom. WL

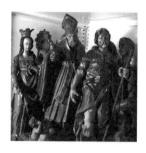

p. 170
Saints in the Science
Museum's Classical and
Mediaeval Medicine
storeroom. WL

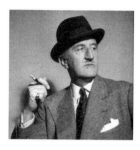

p. 173
Captain Peter Johnston
Johnston-Saint (1886–1974).
WL, V0048809

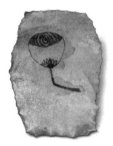

p. 181
Human skin tattooed with
poppy head. French,
1850–1920. SM, A672

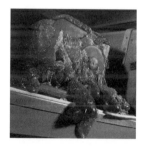

p. 187
Cased inductor coil made by
E. Ducretet, 1870–1910, in
the Science Museum's
Therapeutics storeroom. WL

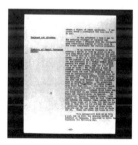

p. 188
Page from Peter Johnston
Johnston-Saint's travel diary,
1 March 1928. Wellcome
Historical Medical Museum
archives.
WA/HMM/RP/JSt/B.2

Acknowledgements

Thanks to Chris Carter, Clive Coward and Kate Darwin in the Wellcome Trust's Photographic Library; to John Symons in the Wellcome Library; and to Stewart Emmens and David Thomas at the Science Museum, all of whom have been exceptionally generous with their time, advice and support.

Permission has been granted for the use of quotations from the following published works:

page 1: 'Things' by Jorge Luis Borges, from *Selected Poems*, edited by Alexander Coleman (Allen Lane The Penguin Press, 1999) reproduced by kind permission of Penguin Books Ltd. Translation copyright © Stephen Kessler, 1999.

page 113: Extract from *Bononbo the Forgotten Ape* by Frans de Waal © 1997, The Regents of the University of California.

page 123: Extract from *The Breast* by Philip Roth, published by Jonathan Cape. Reproduced by permission of The Random House Group Limited.

page 124: Extract from *The Lives of the Gods* by Alberto Savinio. Reproduced by permission of Atlas Press.

Every effort has been made to obtain copyright permission for quoted extracts. Any omissions or errors of attribution are unintentional and will, if brought to the attention of the publisher, be corrected in future printings.